Delivered at Home

DEDICATED TO

the memory of my mother
and
to my sister Jane,
who is also a midwife

Delivered at Home

Julia Allison

Stanley Thornes (Publishers) Ltd

First published by Chapman & Hall in 1996
(ISBN 0 412-56300-2)

Reprinted in 1997 by:
Stanley Thornes (Publishers) Ltd
Ellenborough House
Wellington Street
Cheltenham GL50 1 YW
United Kingdom

97 98 99 00 01 / 10 9 8 7 6 5 4 3 2 1

A catalogue record for this book is available from the British Library

ISBN 0-7487-3500-3

Typeset by Mews Photosetting, Beckenham, Kent
Printed in Great Britain by T.J. International, Padstow, Cornwall

Contents

Foreword

Dame Margaret Brain DBE, RGN, RNT, MTD, FRCOG

I was delighted to be asked to write the foreword for this important book. Soon after I became President of the Royal College of Midwives I met Julia Allison and was immediately impressed by her total commitment to her chosen profession and her obvious love of her work.

Since then I have become enthralled by hearing her speak of her research work which forms the basis of this book. It is a personal testimony.

Midwifery research is still a youthful discipline. Explaining and analysing what midwives do, from a midwife's perspective, is crucial to maintaining the autonomy of our profession and freeing it from the medical and nursing constraints which have tried to bind it. This book is an important contribution to the body of knowledge which tells the real history of midwifery.

Much contemporary research aims to incorporate statistical evidence with social history. This book is in the best of that tradition. It fills the gaps of other research which has demonstrated the safety, effectiveness and responsiveness of midwifery care, by including an account of what it was really like to be a district midwife in the post-war period up until the NHS reorganization of the 1970s. The book will therefore have significance for medical, feminist and social researchers alike, as well as for the midwifery profession as a whole.

Julia has also identified the gaps in her own research and set a challenging research agenda for tomorrow's midwives. There is still much to be told about how women and midwives experienced pregnancy in the days when childbirth belonged firmly in the social/domestic sphere.

This is not an idealized picture of some halcyon past but a realistic account of the strengths and difficulties associated with providing continuity of care to groups of known women. As midwives prepare for the twenty-first century, moving centre stage to reclaim their 'with woman role', there is much that the past can teach about preparing for the future. This book gives an insight into how some of the principles of Changing Childbirth were practised in reality 30 years ago and what exciting and stimulating reading it makes. I am sure its publication will be a milestone for women – as mothers or midwives.

Acknowledgements

The inspiration to train as a midwife came in 1962 when my second child was born at home in Nottingham. He was delivered by one of the midwives in this study. Following district training, working alongside some of these midwives, my career as a domiciliary midwife in Nottingham began towards the end of this period. The experience of domiciliary care as a mother, a student and a colleague of the city midwives, left me with an abiding admiration for their commitment and skills.

I was working on the district in the early 1970s, the time of the implementation of the reorganization of the National Health Service and the Peel Report.

> The changes in professional thought and the administrative action which, it is recommended, should flow from it, must be associated with a change of community attitudes towards midwifery and maternity matters. The obstetric team, which we have indicated as necessary for the service itself, should include among its responsibilities the education of the community to the desirability and benefits of the reorganisation.
>
> *(HMSO 1970)*

While some saw the change as progress, a necessary move in the centralization of specialist functions within the NHS, many of the district midwives felt that the principle upon which their professional belief was founded had shifted. It was painful to witness the crisis of confidence that many endured in trying to come to terms with the fact that home birth with midwife-led care had not only been declared unsafe for mothers and babies, but virtually outlawed. Some who had spent 20 years giving excellent domiciliary care felt that their career was to end in ignominy, and, for them, retirement could not come quickly enough.

This book is dedicated to those midwives, both for their past service to the community and for the generosity with which they gave of their time, records and treasured memories. I have always believed that district midwives have a great untold story; and it is my privilege to share some of it with you.

In the statistical analyses and quotations from interviews, some of the midwives have been mentioned by name. On occasions, some names have been changed for anonymity: where this happens it is noted in the text. Some midwives made very frank and painful disclosures during the interviews and did not wish to be identified although they were happy for their records and interviews to be used. On those occasions, the midwife has simply been described as 'a retired midwife', or some similar description. Similarly, as the registers apply to births which occurred as late as 1972, in discussing cases every effort has been made to ensure that individual midwives or mothers cannot be identified. Nevertheless I wish to put on record my thanks to those midwives and the mothers of Nottingham, without whom this book could not have been written.

An enormous debt of gratitude is owed to so many people: first to the midwives, especially those from the city and county of Nottingham who gave me their time, thoughts, records or memorabilia, to Audrey, Ann, Anne, June (who also spoke for Pat), Edith, Annie, Ruth, Chris (who died in 1991), Barbara, Rosie, Nellie, Olga, Margaret, Brenda, Shirley, Joan, Sue, Sue, Mary, Mary, Gill, Louise, Jackie, Eileen, Constance (now dead, whose daughter allowed me to borrow her register), Dorothy, Doris, Vera, Tilly, Marjorie, Marjorie, Pamela and Joyce. And to the friends and relatives of deceased district midwives, who each gave all the help and information they were able, I offer my thanks.

In addition to those midwives who allowed me to interview them, Olga, who now lives on the Isle of Wight, wrote to me, three long letters full of humour and reminiscences. Where Olga is quoted, the quotations have been taken from her letters, which made a lively contribution to this book.

A special debt of gratitude is owed to Joyce Tarlton, my district teaching midwife and now my friend. Joyce made the biggest single contribution to the archive material: not only has she given her registers, stretching over a 32-year career on the district, but also splendid old textbooks, wartime *Nursing Mirrors,* nursing bags and uniforms and boxes of stationery, letters, minutes of meetings, reports of refresher courses, lists of midwives' names and addresses, old advertising material, and policies and protocols. Joyce is also the amateur photographer who took so many of the evocative photos, including the front cover. Little did she think when she took up photography to give her an interest outside of work, that 30 years later those pictures would be published.

All of Joyce's treasures will finally find a home in the archive planned at the Royal College of Midwives, as will those of the midwives from all over Britain who have sent me textbooks, memorabilia, letters and equipment. I wish to thank them too.

I am indebted to the Department of Health for financial support for a three-month sabbatical, while I was Head of Midwifery Studies in Norfolk, to begin the writing-up process of this research, which has greatly assisted the early completion of this book. Thanks are also due to the obstetricians, midwives, management and administrative staff of Nottingham Health Authority, and Community Unit, during the period 1989–91, who allowed me the time and facility to explore their archives.

I am particularly indebted to Gillian Pascall, Marjorie Tew, Alison Macfarlane, Elizabeth Meerabeau, Gordon Blades, Suzanne Tyler, Kate Jackson, Catherine McCormick and Kathryn Partington for their advice and encouragement. Also to Helen Jessler (who died in 1994), Mary Renfrew, Murray Enkin, Margaret MacIntosh, Rona Campbell, Iain Chalmers, Neville Lees, Jane Robinson, Baroness Julia Cumberlege and Dame Margaret Brain for their encouragement.

I pay tribute to the hospital midwives, obstetricians and general practitioners of the City of Nottingham during the period of the study. Whatever the experiences of the district midwives, they like us were doing the best they knew how, in difficult conditions, to ensure the safety of mothers and babies. Like district midwives, obstetricians were working around the clock; they never failed to support midwives when they were needed and showed great respect for their prowess in normal birth.

Finally, I thank Barrie, for his love and endless cups of coffee during all those evenings when he sat patiently quiet while I tapped away on the lap-top. And our children Melanie and Jon, their partners Alan and Jayne and grandchildren James, Nicholas (delivered at home by grandma), Sophie, Hayley, Hannah and Sasha who are the inspiration of my life and are always a loving support. The book, however, is mine, as is any shortcoming in its form or content.

Introduction

Knowing your past does not automatically yield solutions to the
problems of the present; but without knowledge of the past it would
be impossible even to consider addressing those problems. The
achievements of professional history are staggering; whatever topic
you choose, you'll find there exists a sound body of professional
knowledge.

(Arthur Marwick 1970/1989)

This book is about district midwives, and mothers and babies who were
delivered at home. It is about one short period in the history of midwifery,
a recent time, to which, some would argue, distance has lent enchantment.
This 24-year period began at the implementation of the National Health
Service in 1948 and ended at its reorganization in 1972, just 24 years
during which, in England and Wales, birth took place in hospital under
the supervision of obstetricians, and at home under the supervision of
district midwives in almost equal proportions. However, this book is not
simply about home birth, but about the degree of care that midwives have
given and can give if allowed to get on with the job for which they are
educated.

Today, clear policy direction has been given for a woman-centred
maternity service in which midwives will be lead carers for some women
(HMSO 1993). Questions have been asked about the ability and readiness
of today's midwife to take on the challenge to change the way in which
they provide care. Alarmists continue to question the wisdom, in terms of
maternal and infant safety, of allowing midwives to act as lead carer in a
service that calls for critical analysis, decision-making and the implementation of appropriate action or referral in potentially life-threatening
situations. However, new systems of care are being devised which, once

more, call upon midwives to utilize their skills to the full. The evaluation of these schemes will be an important aspect of the changing maternity service.

It is a matter of regret that the work of district midwives was never properly evaluated; nor were fair outcome comparisons made between home and hospital births, midwife or medically led care. Certain historic assumptions about the risk status of women who were booked for home birth tended to make the widely differing statistical differences explainable in terms of the assumed low-risk status of women delivered at home. The optimum time for making those comparisons has passed. This book tries to reconstruct, as far as the availability of contemporary records will allow, the information available to a researcher of the day, had a fair comparison been attempted. To a great extent district midwives provided midwife-led, woman-centred caré and that care will be contextualized in a contemporary socioeconomic and professional framework.

This book is based on the emerging findings of what is believed to be the only systematic analysis of the work of district midwives. The reader is invited to see it not simply as an exposition of home birth, but for what it says about how midwifery services were organized and run when midwives were the lead carers for 50% of women. That all of these births occurred at home is in one sense academic. We cannot look at a time when 50% of hospital births were under the leadership of a mid-wife because that time has not yet come. What we can learn from this study is about partnership and team midwifery, caseloads, workloads, hours on duty and on call, the outcomes of midwifery-led care and something of our history that is worthy of note. In the era which this book examines, more than 90% of births at home in Nottingham were conducted by the district midwife or pupil with no doctor in attendance. Even on those occasions when a doctor was present s/he seldom conducted the birth.

This introduction describes the aim, data, analysis, methodology and background search, and the structure of the book.

Between 1948 and 1972 in Britain, local authorities provided domicil-iary midwifery services for up to 50% of women: those who gave birth at home. The system changed over time as a consequence of local government reforms (HMSO 1969) and the recommendations of Cranbrook (HMSO 1959) and Peel (HMSO 1970) for increased numbers of women to be confined in hospital. It was finally abandoned at the re-organization of the National Health Service (HMSO 1972); although the demise of an effective domiciliary midwifery service was more to do with the assumption that birth in hospital was safest for all women. Chief among those who have continued to challenge that belief are Rona Campbell and Alison Macfarlane (1987) and Marjorie Tew (1995).

AIM OF THE BOOK

The aim of the book is to describe a retrospective study of the work of district midwives, and the 62 444 home births undertaken by the district midwives of the City of Nottingham between 1948 and 1972. In the light of today's changing maternity services, key questions emerge from within the wider descriptive framework of the book. As health authorities and trusts seek to find new ways of organizing midwifery services to meet the challenge of offering 'woman-centred care', how in comparison, did district midwifery work, in terms of organization and caseload? Similarly, to what extent could their work be described as team midwifery and what level of success was achieved in providing continuity of carer and choice?

In the continuing debate about the place of birth and the safety of mothers and babies to deliver anywhere other than a consultant maternity unit, other questions arise. What were the criteria and selection processes for home birth? What were the transfer rates and what were the outcomes of home delivery in terms of the safety of mother and baby and client satisfaction?

These issues will be revisited in the final chapters and, drawing upon the text, an attempt will be made to evaluate the relevance of the way in which district midwives worked to today's changing maternity services.

THE INVESTIGATION

The approach to this research developed as data became available; what started as a small study to look at the registers of three district midwives for evidence of outcomes to babies born at home before the arrival of the midwife (BBAs), grew as more data became available. The search, begun in 1989, was focused in Nottingham and drew upon my own experience as a district midwife.

The birth registers of city midwives with whom I had worked were collected together, my own included. This involved an informal visit to each midwife's home, at which notes were taken of her recollections in an unstructured interview. Not every midwife had her registers: some had been handed in to the local authority when they retired or moved, some had been destroyed in a flood at Perth Street, Health Department office. No city midwife declined to let me have her registers, if they were in her possession. In the course of tracing the midwives I sometimes spoke to their friends or relatives to find that the midwife had died. Friends and relatives endeavoured to give me as much help as possible in tracing their registers and generously shared their memories.

The Director of Nottingham Health Authority Community Unit and the Community Supervisor of Midwives gave me permission to search the community archives and borrow any material which was germane to the investigation. I found two sets of registers of long retired city midwives, which I borrowed in 1990, entered into the computer and returned to the archive in 1991. In the 1960s there had been a flood at the Health Department offices at Perth Street, Nottingham, in which all of the midwifery archive material stored there was lost. This included the personal registers of retired district midwives who had chosen to hand them in to the Supervisor of Midwives.

During the course of the initial visits to the midwives the names of other midwives were given and from that information it was possible to trace more. Inevitably some of the midwives are dead and two were too ill to talk to me. Most of the midwives gave me additional material, including a great deal of memorabilia, photographs, letters, certificates, uniforms and equipment and official lists of city midwives, which further helped the inquiry. As interest in my research grew, retired district midwives began to contact me and in this way I collected data from Nottingham county midwives and some from other areas. On completion of my studies, all the material and data gifted to me will be given to the Royal College of Midwives, where an archive for future readers and researchers is being planned. Other material has been returned to the midwives who so kindly lent it to me for the purpose of this study.

During 1990 and 1991 a number of semi-structured interviews were undertaken with ten retired city midwives. These included questions about their workload, professional relationships, training, personal life and their perception of their status as a district midwife. Each had very individual stories to tell and I quickly learned that if the discussion was structured too tightly there was a danger of missing important information. I carried out all the interviews, and also interviewed two retired general practitioner obstetricians, two retired non-medical Supervisors of Midwives and two premature baby midwives.

No investigation of this nature could ever be said to be complete, and I am aware that there were some midwives who were never reached and some stones that were left unturned. However, in 1994 after five years' search it was time to draw the investigation to a conclusion and to make use of what had been collected. From the enormous amount of data and memorabilia, for the purpose of this book two particular sources have been used.

CITY OF NOTTINGHAM DISTRICT MIDWIVES' PERSONAL REGISTERS

During the time of the search it was possible to trace 54 personal registers of 14 district midwives, detailing births, 19% of home births in the city in the period. They contain a contemporaneous record of every delivery undertaken by each individual midwife. The registers represent home births in every part of the city. Two of the midwives worked exclusively, and throughout most of the period of the study, on the large council housing estate being built at that time in south Nottingham. The majority of deliveries occurred in the inner city area and six large council estates to the north of the city. The remaining registers include births in all those areas, for some or all of the period. Thus it can be said that the registers represent in some way, a spread across the whole city, though it is unlikely that they are an absolutely representative sample.

Each of the midwives worked at some time during the period 1948–72, some beginning their district career before 1948 and some completing it after 1972. Between them they gave 222 years service. Seven of the midwives undertook between 700 and 1000 home births and two achieved a total of around 2000.

The style and form of the personal registers, which were supplied through the Central Midwives Board (CMB) and became the property of the midwife, changed over time. The most radical change took place in the 1950s when the register lost its traditional tall shape with ten entries on a double page and took on the now familiar modern shape with six entries per double page. At that time the information recorded at birth was extended to include the date of the booking, the name of the GP booked for maternity medical services, and the name of any doctor present or called to the birth, the birthweight, the method of feeding at discharge and the drugs given. Therefore not all the information that is available from registers today is available for the whole of the period. Several other changes were made to the registers over the years but none that radically affected this data analysis. The information listed below can be gleaned from all the modern registers and most, but not all, from the traditional registers and includes:

- name, address, age and parity of client;
- name of GP, if booked;
- GP called in emergency;
- date of booking;
- estimated date of delivery (EDD);
- antenatal care given by;
- date and time of midwife's arrival at delivery;
- name of person performing delivery;
- other professional persons present at delivery;
- date and time of birth and weight of baby;
- baby – alive or dead/abnormalities;
- whether transferred to hospital – mother and/or baby;
- condition of mother and baby on discharge;

- method of feeding and weight at discharge
- drugs given in labour, at birth and immediate postnatal period;
- type of delivery, e.g. prolonged labour, presentation, multiple birth;
- medical aid or flying squad called;
- medical treatment required, e.g. transfusion, drugs, resuscitation.

ANNUAL HEALTH SERVICE REPORTS OF THE MEDICAL OFFICER OF HEALTH FOR THE CITY OF NOTTINGHAM, 1948–72

Contents include the following information/statistics:

- home and hospital births;
- stillbirths, perinatal deaths and maternal deaths by cause and place of birth;
- premature births by weight of infant, place of birth and outcome;
- number of midwives, domiciliary, hospital, private practice;
- number of medical aid calls to maternity cases;
- number of times GPs present at births;
- legitimacy of babies;
- number of times emergency obstetric team called by cause;
- details of midwives' workloads and conditions;
- work of premature baby midwives;
- various information such as level of antenatal care to women who had a stillbirth;
- annual analysis of the work of the supervisor of midwives;
- continuing education programmes of district midwives;
- allocation of district pupils and medical students.

Throughout the period these annual reports routinely contained comprehensive data related to the work of the district midwife, supervision, home and hospital births, stillbirths and maternal deaths. Other data collected for national statistical returns, such as information about low birthweight babies, was published from time to time. In 1968 the data was modified and by 1972 the standard of data collection and analysis had deteriorated. After 1972 they were no longer published.

In addition to these two main sources, selected oral evidence, photographs and other archive material has been used.

THE SOCIETY AND RESIDENTS OF THE CITY OF NOTTINGHAM

During the time in question and prior to the Local Government Act 1969, Nottingham was the eighth largest city in England, with a population of

312 000. It is upon the births to residents, and the work of district midwives of the City of Nottingham, that the research is focused.

In terms of social, economic and industrial variety, Nottingham shared similar experiences to other large industrial cities of the time. It was the subject of post-war slum clearance, housing shortage, overcrowding and latterly the much despised high-rise flats. In the 1950/60s immigrants from the West Indies were heavily represented in the statistics for mothers seeking hospital birth on the grounds of poor social conditions. Nottingham's industries included coal-mining, cigarette and cycle manufacture and a manufacturing chemist. There was little unemployment in the years in question. Working-class women tended to be employed in the cigarette, hosiery or lace-making trades.

One strength of using data from Nottingham is that home birth remained as a viable alternative to hospital birth for many years longer than the national average. While working towards the government policy to hospitalize childbirth, Nottingham was hampered by a shortage of maternity beds, which was not addressed until the opening of the Nottingham City hospital maternity unit in 1973. Thus while the home-birth rate had diminished by 1957 to 35.4% of births nationally (Towler and Bramall 1986: 252), it remained at more than 50% of total births in the City of Nottingham until 1963; even in 1972 it was 21%. This gives an opportunity to make comparisons between home- and hospital-birth outcomes into the 1970s.

Another reason for using this data is the number of research studies which were undertaken in Nottingham regarding home birth, maternity care and social aspects of childbearing and rearing. More than twenty were traced, many of a substantive nature; some were commissioned by the health authority, some were published across the world. Foremost among them is John and Elizabeth Newson, *Patterns of Infant Care in an Urban Community*, first published in 1963. Equally useful was the medical thesis of John Goodacre (1974), *A Survey of Home and Hospital Confinements in Nottingham*.

Local authorities provided domiciliary midwifery services for home birth across Britain at this time but they were not a mirror image of each other. LAs had autonomy in deciding how these services would be provided within the statutory framework and decisions were largely dependent upon the level of provision of hospital and private maternity care, and the demography and geography of the area they served. In that regard the City of Nottingham domiciliary midwifery service could not be said to be truly representative of every domiciliary midwifery service in Britain. City, county and borough services throughout the country differed but most gave midwives a geographically linked caseload, at least for the greater part of the study.

Differences between city and county services were mainly due to the local geography. Whereas city midwives might have small, tightly spaced patches and caseloads, county midwives, especially in rural counties such as Norfolk, Somerset, Devon and Yorkshire, frequently found that even with a large 'patch' the number of childbearing women in any year would not sustain a district midwive's post; thus domiciliary services were provided by double or triple duty nurses/workers (see Appendix B, Glossary, page 139).

Throughout the latter period, Nottingham, like Liverpool, also suffered that type of inner-city poverty and growth in racial disharmony which led to race riots in the city in the 1970s. In certain ways Nottingham could be said to represent a picture of some of the extreme social circumstances prevailing in Britain during the period in question.

THE ERA 1948–1972

The era began as the Second World War ended and Britain struggled to recover from the effects of bomb damage and loss of life. There was an employment crisis as thousands of men returned from overseas to find no job in 'civvy street'. Local authorities implemented plans to rebuild slum- and bomb-damaged houses and to provide thousands of temporary prefabricated council houses. The National Health Service began in 1947, as did the baby boom following the return of servicemen from abroad.

During this time ownership of a family car slowly became the norm. Homes which at the beginning of the period had only a copper in which to boil the weekly wash were later equipped with a washing machine and a growing range of modern labour-saving machines. Women who in the late 1940s were fully occupied as housewives were now taking their place in the work-force, undertaking higher education and entering the professions and management. The average number of children in the family declined as a national family-planning programme got underway.

As this period ended there was an economic boom, jobs were plentiful and home ownership was an achievable objective for most who were determined to have their own home. The National Health Service had been a good servant during the long post-war struggle and was about to undergo its first reorganization.

The Christian Dior 'New Look' of the late 1940s, the mini-skirt of the 1960s, the flares and platform shoes of the 1970s: the fashions were reflected in the uniforms of the district midwives. From the formal uniform of the 1950s midwife (page xxi), to the peep at the midwife's knee in a near mini-skirted uniform dress of the 1960s (page 18), even district midwives tried to keep abreast of fashion.

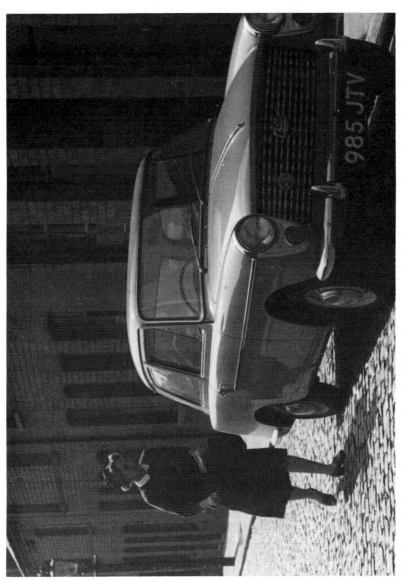

District midwife and transport in the 1960s. (Reproduced with kind permission from Joyce Tarlton.)

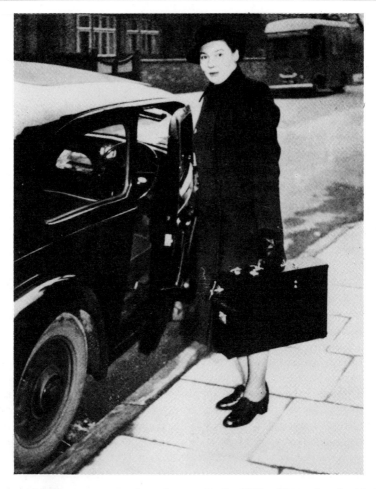

District midwife transport and equipment in the 1960s. (Reproduced with kind permission from the MOH.)

DATA ANALYSIS

All data from Annual Medical Officer of Health Reports related to domiciliary and hospital births have been entered into a 'Works' programme on an Apple Macintosh computer, as has information on stillbirths, multiple pregnancies, BBAs and 'risk' factors. Information from midwives' registers was coded for anonymity and entered into a Statistical Package for Social Sciences (SPSS) program. In the following chapters the reader will note that the time span for statistical tables differs between topics under discussion. In all cases all available data has been used. The different time spans are due to the limits of data collection and publication by the Medical Officer of Health, or of the availability of information from the registers.

An attempt was made to ensure that the entire data was entered for future researchers, before the registers were returned to their owners. However, neither the time nor resources could be found and those registers which were loaned from midwives have now been returned. Each midwife has been asked to consider bequeathing her registers to the Royal College of Midwives' archive.

BACKGROUND SEARCH

The background search included examination of statutory instruments and government and professional body reports, and reports and literature related to Nottingham to provide data and professional, political and social background. Although no previous systematic analysis of the work of district midwives is thought to have been attempted, and in that sense this research is peculiar, there are themes within the study to which other researchers and writers have made inspiring contributions: namely, the debate about place of birth and carer.

Marjorie Tew was the first to challenge the assumption that birth in hospital was safest for all women. Tew claims that the medical profession propagated the belief that the decline in maternal and infant deaths over the past 50 years was due to the increased management of birth in hospital by obstetricians (Tew 1978, 1979, 1986). Her impartial examination of the statistical, observational and biological evidence points to the reverse conclusion. Her hypothesis is that safety in childbirth depends on the good health of mothers brought about by rising standards of living and nutrition. Her contribution which began in the 1970s was elaborated in her 1990 publication *Safer Childbirth* (Tew second edn. 1995).

The most relevant literature in regard to this study is the work of Campbell and MacFarlane (1987, reprinted 1994) *Where to be Born, the Debate and the Evidence*, in crystallizing the issues about place of birth and highlighting the anonymity of the midwife both in statistics and evidence. Their analysis, which examined all available evidence about the merits of the different places of birth, questioned the extent to which policies about where women gave birth were related to available evidence. Among their conclusions were the following:

- The statistical association between the increase in the proportion of hospital deliveries and the fall in the crude perinatal mortality rate seems unlikely to be explained by a cause-and-effect relation.

- The rise in the crude perinatal mortality rate for births at home can almost certainly be explained by the increase in the proportion of unplanned births at home relative to those planned to occur there: a consequence of the fall in the overall number of home births.
- The Home Births Survey showed perinatal mortality among births to the select group of women who had planned deliveries at home to be very low, particularly among parous women.
- There is no evidence to support the claim that the safe policy is for all women to give birth in hospital.
- A majority of women who experienced both home and hospital deliveries prefer to have their babies at home, although this may include a disproportionate number of women who have sought home delivery after a hospital delivery with which they were dissatisfied.

Campbell and MacFarlane's contribution has been a powerful influence in changing the political attitude towards the place of birth, the role of the midwife and women's choice.

This research gives an added dimension to many of the discussions and conclusions reached by Tew, Campbell and Macfarlane. In particular it brings the role of the district midwife as lead carer at home deliveries into focus. Most previous studies have viewed birth in terms of obstetrician or GP cases; here we will see the outcomes of tens of thousands of home births where, in terms of giving the majority of antenatal care, predominance as sole carer at the birth and being the only provider of postnatal care, the district midwife becomes the evident lead carer for women who had home births in Nottingham between 1948 and 1972.

In addition, assumptions that women who were booked for home birth were a carefully selected group of women in the 'low risk' category will be shown to be flawed; in reality at least 50% of women who gave birth at home during the period of the study in Nottingham did not fulfil the criteria for home birth. Tew (1985: 390), in discussing the unpublished results of the 1970 *British Birth* survey, highlights the fact that by the time of the survey 66% of births (nationally) were taking place in consultant units with a hospital perinatal death rate of 27.8 per 1000 compared to the home birth perinatal death rate of 4.3 per 1000. She further discloses that not only was this disparity not discussed, neither was any evidence presented that might have shown that the higher perinatal mortality rate in hospital was due to a greater rate of high risk cases.

Probably the most complex but revealing element of this research is the work and discussion about the number of transfers in and out of domiciliary care. The long held belief, which was central to a policy for 100% hospital birth, is that the transfer of women from home to hospital was a one-way phenomenon, causing hospital mortality outcomes to be adversely skewed by the number of cases originally booked for home but later transferred to hospital care. However, by examining evidence from Nottingham it becomes clear that, within this research, it is likely that while some women were transferred from home to hospital in labour, a greater number who were hospital booked or unbooked, having had no antenatal care were finally delivered at home.

The book uses elements of the historical data, interviews and archive material to place on record something of the statistical outcomes, professional, social and domestic history of district midwives and the mothers and babies they served. It is structured in the following way:

CHAPTER ONE: THE WORK AND LIFE OF DISTRICT MIDWIVES

This chapter seeks to explain some of the key features of Nottingham's domiciliary midwifery service and the work of its district midwives, which were a reflection, though not a mirror image, of local authority domiciliary midwifery services offered across Britain. First the organization, management and personnel who comprised the district-based domiciliary midwifery service are described. This reveals that domiciliary midwifery services were provided by a discrete district-based service, whose chief executive and all senior staff, which included the Supervisors of Midwives, were required to have a midwifery, maternity service and public health background.

The training, working arrangements, caseloads and workloads of district midwives are also discussed, together with the midwives' relationship to general practitioners, obstetricians and local authority clinics, families and colleagues. Evidence that the workloads of district midwives were too great, that caseloads were too high and not fairly distributed will be shown, as will the midwives' view of their own self-esteem and their high regard in the public eye. What becomes evident is that many of the domiciliary midwives chose to train and work on the district as a career for life. The appointment and grade of district midwives, their marital status, role as teacher of midwifery and medical students and premature baby midwife are among the other issues examined in this chapter.

The way in which district midwives worked in Nottingham changed over time due to the implementation of early discharge from hospital and introduction of a night rota system; this affected the level of continuity of care for some women. The working arrangements of the district midwives are described in two phases. Phase One covers the period 1947–64 and Phase Two 1965–72.

Some attempt is made to look at the professional life of the district midwife in Nottingham, in the context of her social and domestic existence. One thing becomes evident: that in the early period in question the delineation between the two is hard to find.

CHAPTER TWO: CHOOSING THE PLACE OF BIRTH

In this chapter issues central to determining where women gave birth in Nottingham during the period of the study are discussed; in consequence, the familiar argument that women who were delivered at home were low risk for complication, loses its impact.

First, the places of birth and types of maternity carer available in Nottingham are described. Second, the criteria which were applied to women and their circumstances to decide where their baby would be born, and to what extent women in Nottingham fulfilled those criteria are deliberated. Last, the extent to which women were selected or able to choose their place of birth or carer is discussed, and the extent to which these systems of care offered continuity of carer are explored.

It becomes evident that because of maternity bed shortage, district midwives delivered at home not only women who chose home birth but also those who could not be fitted into the system elsewhere. Further, that in addition to selection by home birth criteria, there was a secondary selection system for hospital birth which had as much to do with social class as it did with obstetric criteria.

CHAPTER THREE: TRANSFERS IN AND OUT OF DOMICILIARY CARE

In this chapter the extent to which home-booked women in Nottingham were transferred to hospital care antenatally and in labour is examined. Conversely, the extent to which hospital-booked and unbooked women were delivered at home and counted in home birth statistics is also examined.

For the past 30 years there has been a belief that, during the period of the study, the transfer of care between home and hospital was a one-way phenomenon which caused hospital outcomes alone to be unfavourably skewed by the high mortality of cases originally booked for home but later transferred to hospital care (Butler and Bonham 1963: 288). City of Nottingham data reveals that this is not as straight-forward as was assumed. Indeed it is evident from this study that it is likely that more unbooked and hospital-booked women, with their high perinatal mortality risk, were unintentionally delivered at home than home-booked women were transferred to hospital in labour. Further, that while the antenatal transfer of women to obstetric care in the ante-natal period was 8.6% of total home bookings, the number of women transferred from home to hospital in labour was only 1.1% of total home births.

Had the data produced by the Supervisors of Midwives and published by the Medical Officers of Health been effectively analysed and presented during the period in question, it is doubtful that the case for 100% hospital births on the grounds of safety could have been upheld.

CHAPTER FOUR: HOME CONFINEMENT – OUTCOMES AND EXPERIENCES

Until recently, birth at home was part of the culture of British society. In this chapter we explore, in statistical terms, the outcomes to mother and baby of home delivery. The provision of social services was not so much a consumer-led function as it is today and assessing to what extent women were satisfied with the domiciliary midwifery care they received is more problematical than assessing the statistical evidence. However, an attempt is made to describe preparation for home delivery from the mothers' perspective and such evidence as there is regarding consumer opinion will be drawn upon.

In the last analysis it is the evaluation of systems of care which should determine the way in which they are maintained or changed over time. What is not in doubt is that home birth as an alternative to hospital birth would not have been effectively outlawed by the 1980s if consumer opinion had been a central plank in policy-making for the provision of maternity services, as it is in the 1990s.

Statistical outcomes of midwifery care in the City of Nottingham 1948–72 are discussed, including maternal death and stillbirth at home and hospital. Interesting disclosures include the fact that the majority of stillbirths occurring at home were to women who were not booked for home confinement. Similarly, in the case of unattended births at home, the majority who sustained a stillbirth were to unbooked or hospital-booked women. Nevertheless the overall outcomes at home were good.

Other aspects of maternity care which are examined include the use of oxygen at birth by district midwives, the incidence of multiple birth at home and the care and outcomes of low birthweight babies at home and hospital. Some new light is shed upon the incidence of breast-feeding in home-delivered mothers, which shows that there was outcome variation between individual midwives.

The outcomes of birth at home, read in the context of the number of women who did not fulfil the criteria for home delivery, and those who were unbooked or booked for hospital, and counted in home-birth statistics confirm the inadequacy of the evidence upon which the policy to move towards 100% hospital birth was made.

CHAPTER FIVE: LEARNING THE LESSONS OF THE PAST

In this chapter we return to the questions posed in the Introduction, and summarize and draw together the findings about how district midwifery worked in terms of organization and caseload. Similarly we discuss to what extent their work could be described as team midwifery and what level of success was achieved in providing continuity of carer and choice.

In terms of the continuing debate about the place of birth, an attempt is made to see to what extent this study contributes to that argument. What were the criteria and selection processes for home birth? What were the transfer rates and what were the outcomes of home delivery in terms of the safety of mother and baby and client satisfaction?

In reality, both the criteria and selection processes proved to be arbitrary, while the transfer rates of home-booked women in the ante-natal period was 8.6% and in labour 1.1%, even though 52% of women who delivered at home did not fulfil the criteria for a home birth. The maternal and infant mortality rates can best be described as comparatively good.

CHAPTER SIX: MIDWIVES AND THE FUTURE MATERNITY SERVICES

Health authorities and trusts are seeking to find new ways of organizing midwifery services to meet the challenge of offering 'woman-centred care'. The purpose of this chapter is to examine the findings of this study of the work of district midwives in Nottingham and to see if they have any relevance for today's midwife. In this final chapter, some issues that arise out of the study are discussed in relation to today's changing maternity services: the education of midwives in preparation for giving 'woman-centred care', our relationship with medical colleagues, the concepts of team approaches to midwifery care and caseloads,. The grade and status of midwives is contemplated in relation to the findings of the study.

At Appendix C some indication is given of the questions that could be asked of the data, yet unexamined, which will eventually be put in the Royal College of Midwives' archive for future researchers.

In the past it has largely been impossible to separate and analyse the contribution of midwives to maternity care. Research has tended to be obstetrician led, and the collection of data has been medically oriented. Interpretation of research, the driving force behind changing maternity care policy, has inevitably been influenced by the philosophies and practices of the researchers, which in turn has led the role of the midwife being made anonymous. This book is about making midwives visible in research terms in regard to their past and future contribution to the maternity service.

CONTEXT OF THE WRITING

No systematic attempt has been made to modernize the language and terminology of the period, except where it is necessary for the reader to be able to contextualize the discussion in terms of today's language or values. In the period in question, postnatal visits were usually referred to as 'nursings' (see Appendix A page 133), and the postnatal period was statutorily referred to as 'the lying-in period'. When speaking of the number of women she had booked, a district midwife would talk about her 'bookings', seldom her caseload and individual women would be referred to as 'patients' or mothers. The term 'home birth' was never used: all reference to birth at home was either home 'delivery' or most often 'home confinement' (see home confinement form page 78). District midwives were known to their 'patients' as 'nurse' or by their proper formal name, e.g. Mrs Brown (see Chapter One page 36). Some of these phrases are an anathema to today's midwife and when talking to some of the long retired midwives the issue of reference to midwives as 'nurse' and women as 'patients' was raised. Those who retired before 1972 found the semantic arguments puzzling, as one put it:

> We knew who we were and mothers knew who we were ... I can't see what the problem is ... things have changed a lot since my day ... midwives seem more like doctors to me now.

One of the difficulties for a midwife who is writing a book about midwifery is that of language and professional jargon. When a midwife writes and thinks she does so in professional terminology, it is as difficult for us to express ourselves in layman's terms as it is for the layman to understand our jargon. For me to write 'the sterile towel placed under the mother's buttocks at delivery', instead of 'the accouchement sheet' or 'complications after the baby was born and around the time the placenta was delivered', instead of 'complications of the third stage', would seem false. Therefore as the book is about midwives, written by a midwife, I have decided to use the appropriate terminology, making sure wherever possible that the meaning is explicit within the text. Appendix B contains a comprehensive Glossary which I hope lay readers will find useful.

The book has been called *Delivered at Home* for a number of reasons. It was a term widely used by midwives of the day. At booking they would enquire, 'Were your other children delivered at home?' When reporting a new delivery to a colleague they would say 'Mrs Smith was delivered at home last night'. When women spoke to each other they would ask about a new baby 'was s/he delivered at home?'. In another sense this is a mischievous title as one could argue that in being 'delivered at home', some of these women were 'delivered' from the difficulties of a hospital birth.

The work and life of district midwives

In this chapter the work and lives of district midwives are put under the microscope. Their time is seen by some as the 'golden era' of midwifery; others would say differently. This 24-year period from 1948 to 1972 saw many changes in midwives' pay, conditions of service and working hours, in addition to those within their social and domestic lives and career expectations. There is no professional or vocational parallel for the way in which they lived and worked. Domiciliary midwifery was then an entirely female profession, giving a 24-hour a day, 365-day a year, door-to-door service to an entirely female clientele. Working from their own home and accountable only to the Supervisor of Midwives and the client, it is sometimes difficult to see where their professional life ended and their domestic life began. Figure 1.1 shows a district midwife on duty in 1948.

This chapter seeks to explain some of the key features of Nottingham's domiciliary midwifery service and the work of its district midwives. The 1948 Rushcliffe Committee Report introduced the term 'District Midwife'. This was to replace terms previously used for this category of midwife, which were domiciliary midwife, county midwife, borough midwife and municipal midwife. The organization, management and personnel who comprised the district-based domiciliary midwifery service form the framework upon which the work and life of these midwives was built. The training, working arrangements, caseloads and workloads of district midwives are among many features which are discussed in order to give substance and texture to their day-to-day working life. Aspects of their social and domestic existence are revealed, together with their professional relationship to general practitioner obstetricians, obstetricians and local authority clinics. Finally, the appointment and grade of the district midwife, her role as teacher and premature baby midwife and her perception of her status in society are examined.

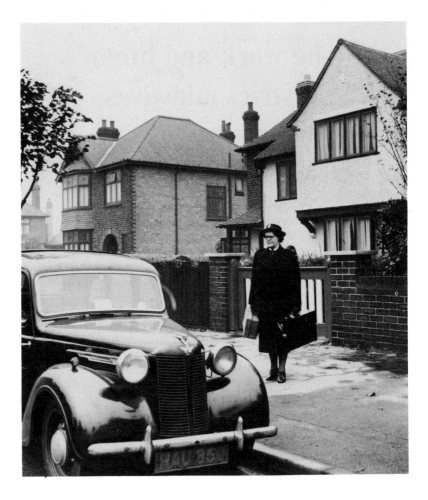

Figure 1.1 The beginning of an era: a district midwife *c.* 1948.

DEVELOPMENT OF LOCAL AUTHORITY DOMICILIARY MIDWIFERY SERVICES

Under Section 103 of the Local Government Act 1933, the Medical Officer of Health was appointed as the chief executive officer of the local authority (Carter and Dodd 1953: 614), otherwise known as local government. He had to be a registered medical practitioner holding a registered diploma in public health, or its equivalent, and he was required to present an annual report to the council. The 1936 Midwives Act placed responsibility on local supervising authorities to provide domiciliary midwives. Domiciliary midwifery services fell within the scope of the health committees of public health departments. In addition to his responsibility to provide a domiciliary midwifery service, the Medical Officer of Health also managed public housing, local social services, education, maternal and child health and other services generally described as 'public health'. Thus domiciliary midwives provided a community-based service which interfaced with other functions of 'public health' affecting the well-being of families. Similarly, public health departments were district based and not allied to acute hospital services.

The National Health Service Act 1946, Section 23, made the local health authority the supervising authority under the Midwives Act. It stated that every local health authority, whether by arrangement with the board of governors of teaching hospitals, hospital management committees or voluntary organizations, or by employing midwives itself, had a duty to employ certificated midwives. It further stated that the number of certificated midwives available for attendance on women in their homes, as midwives, or as maternity nurses during childbirth and the lying-in period, should be adequate for the needs of the area. Nothing in the Act prevented a midwife from practising independently, but her fees would not be included in the free service provided under the National Health Service Act (Carter and Dodds 1953: 636).

Under Section 22 of the NHS Act 1946, medical officers provided medical maternity care at local authority antenatal clinics, which were also attended by district midwives. MOs were generally required to have been qualified for three years and to have adequate experience of practical midwifery and antenatal work. Nottingham's local authority employed four medical officers.

Supervision of midwives was carried out by the local health authority, acting as the local supervising authority, and exercised by the Medical Officer of Health or any person appointed by him for the purpose. A non-medical supervisor had to be in active practice as a midwife for a minimum of three years, with one year's district experience.

For the period of the study the City of Nottingham had one full-time non-medical Supervisor of Midwives and an assistant full-time non-medical

Supervisor of Midwives, both employed within the district midwifery team and based in the Health Department, reporting directly to the Medical Officer of Health. The Medical Officer of Health served as the Medical Supervisor. Supervision of midwives was zealously carried out and to a great extent it is the work and records of supervisors which have facilitated the production of this history.

In effect, the functional and executive management structure of the domiciliary midwifery service was entirely composed of personnel with qualification and proven expertise in maternity care. Furthermore, the entire focus and location of domiciliary midwifery services was district-based with no functional, financial or executive control from hospital-based services.

DISTRICT MIDWIVES: TRAINING AND QUALIFICATIONS (NATIONAL PERSPECTIVE)

When statutory training began in 1902, midwifery was a profession mainly taught and practised in the home; following entry to the roll, a midwife was able to put up her plate and practise in her neighbourhood. It could be argued that district midwives were the last of this tradition.

In the time of this study, women with no nursing qualification (direct entrants) undertook eighteen months Part 1 training and six months Part 2, of which a minimum of three months was spent 'on the district'. Women with a nursing qualification usually undertook six months Part 1 and Part 2 training (CMB 1950).

A 1963 survey (Mason 1963) showed that direct entrants were usually older women whose families were complete; the majority were employed as district midwives immediately after training. There is no evidence, either in the literature search or in the findings of this research, that the quality of work of newly qualified district midwives was different from that of midwives who had practised for longer. Similarly there is no evidence that the quality of work differed between direct entrants and midwives who held a nursing qualification.

The report also showed that one year after qualification 75% of direct entrants in the study remained in practice compared to 47% of (nurse) midwives.

QUALIFICATIONS OF CITY OF NOTTINGHAM DISTRICT MIDWIVES

From training school records and oral evidence it is clear that while many City of Nottingham midwives held a nursing qualification, an equal number were direct entrants. This is interesting as the number of nurses who qualified as midwives was far in excess of the number of direct entrants. While there was one intake of five direct entrants, there were several intakes of 12 pupil midwives who were nurse qualified each year. During interview, all the five direct entrant retired district midwives revealed that their sole reason for undertaking midwifery training was to practise as a domiciliary midwife. Each of them took up post immediately they qualified and none of them practised anywhere other than the district.

One direct entry midwife said:

> I trained to be a midwife and look after women ... three children of my own and lots of friends with kids. I understood what women wanted ... I didn't train to dance round after a man [meaning doctors] ...I'd got one at home ... I didn't jump round after him ... I wasn't going in hospital to do it ... if I thought it would have helped women or saved babies I would have ... although perhaps I'd never have trained, perhaps I'd have let some-one else get on with it.

It is worth noting that this midwife adapted her practice to undertake domino births when they were introduced.

Those who held a nursing qualification prior to undertaking midwifery training (five) had less focused reasons for undertaking midwifery, four held a hospital midwifery post before entering the domiciliary service and all five stayed on the district until they retired.

Joyce, one of the nurse-trained midwives, gave a total service of 32 years, although shortly after entering service as a district midwife she undertook the premature baby course and worked for several years as one of the premature baby midwives before returning to work as a district midwife.

One of the factors which influenced direct entry midwives' choice of career path was the fact that women accepted into direct entry training in Nottingham were generally required to have a minimum of five 'O' levels, a rare occurrence in those days, and to be mature with suitable life's experience, normally interpreted as married with children aged over ten years. Such women could be expected to have a clear notion of what they wanted to achieve in career terms, which would be more likely to embrace the opportunity to practise with professional independence and social flexibility. Also, direct entrants only had one qualification and did not have an option to return to nursing.

Author's note: In the direct entry intake in which I trained there were three local candidates, including myself. We each took a district post on qualification. Jean remained on the district until she retired in the 1980s. Anne still works on the community and continues to undertake home births for women who request them. I finally resigned my community post in 1985 to be a midwife teacher.

Those who entered following nurse training were usually younger, less likely to be domestically tied and frequently undertook midwifery training as a means to gaining a second certificate, rather than from an initial desire to be a midwife. Two certificates were often a prerequisite to getting a sister's post either in nursing or midwifery and to entering training as a health visitor.

In addition to direct entry and entry as a state registered nurse, there were other forms of shortened programme: for example, it was possible for a state enrolled nurse to train as a midwife if she fulfilled the educational requirements.

WORKING ARRANGEMENTS AND CONTINUITY OF CARE

The way in which district midwives worked in Nottingham changed over time due to the implementation of early discharge from hospital and the introduction of a night rota system; this affected the level of continuity of care for some women. The working arrangements are described in two phases.

PHASE ONE: 1947–64

City midwives worked in partnerships of two or three, each midwife caring for women in a geographic patch; her partner/s practised in adjacent patches. They kept each other informed about their clients and by the end of the 1950s held a weekly joint clinic where women met each midwife in the partnership.

The majority of women saw no more than three or four carers throughout the whole childbearing experience; midwife and partner, GP and perhaps a pupil midwife or medical student. Some who did not book a GP saw only their midwife. Women were guaranteed continuity of carer. The registers of two midwives who worked in partnership show that all of the 420 women (excluding any hospital and unbooked cases) delivered by them during 1958 and 1959 were booked with them for home birth.

During this time, city midwives were primarily engaged in the care of women booked for home birth, while women booked for hospital birth were cared for by hospital maternity carers, who similarly guaranteed them a high level of continuity of carer (Allison 1991: 32–35).

PHASE TWO: 1965–72

For six years city midwives resisted requests by the MOH to adopt a night-rota scheme, despite the fact that it would reduce the number of occasions on which they were on call. They were concerned that women would be looked after in labour by a stranger and that the thick fogs which prevailed in Nottingham in the 1960s might prevent a midwife finding an unfamiliar address (City of Nottingham 1960: 28).

It is worth noting that at this time midwives were paid a salary for the job; they were not paid an 'on call' allowance or unsocial hours. Thus it could be argued that their reasons for resisting a change that would reduce the number of occasions on which they had a broken night's sleep were truly altruistic.

In 1965 a night-rota system was introduced against the wishes of the midwives (City of Nottingham 1965: 33). Each night, seven midwives were on call throughout the city attending births wherever they occurred. This reduced the number of times a midwife was on call and the client's chance of a known carer at delivery. At the same time, the increasing numbers of early discharges from hospital further fragmented the midwife's work as she developed two systems of care: one for home bookings and one for hospital-booked clients. A high level of continuity of carer for home-booked women was maintained, but could no longer be guaranteed. No continuity of carer could be offered to women who were booked for hospital birth; they shared antenatal care with the GP, the obstetrician and the district midwife, and were eventually delivered by an unknown midwife in the maternity unit.

CASELOADS, DELIVERIES AND WORKLOAD

A caseload was the number of women booked for delivery with a district midwife in a year. The number of women actually delivered did not necessarily correspond with her caseload, as some were attended by her partner and vice versa. However, midwives who had the largest caseloads almost inevitably had the largest workloads. From oral evidence and the midwives' registers, it can be seen that midwives who delivered partners' cases frequently continued with the postnatal care, at the request of the woman. Women often showed a preference for continuity from the midwife who had delivered their baby, who they would already know, demonstrating that the carer at delivery was particularly important to the woman. Indeed, this midwife had shared in a most intimate event in a family's life.

The 1949 Rushcliffe working party recommended a caseload of no more than 55 women per annum for an urban midwife (Carter and Dodds 1953). In 1963, the average caseload of city midwives was 106 (City of Nottingham 1963: 32). The caseloads of city midwives, on average, were far above the recommendations of Rushcliffe from the inception of the service until 1970. The situation, which was reflected in hospital, was due to a chronic national shortage of midwives; the medical officer of health reported that he was constantly striving to bring staff levels to that required by the Rushcliffe Committee.

One difficulty of providing caseload care is uneven work spread. Many attempts were made to address this problem, including the use of district registers to record bookings across an area. From time to time, geographic patches were redefined to give more cases to one midwife and less to another. This was often thwarted by midwives who continued to book every woman who approached them; oral evidence of a Supervisor of Midwives reveals that one midwife delivered in excess of 200 women for several years in succession in the 1950s. However, she did not wish to accept help with her workload as her caseload consisted in the main of women she had known for many years and did not wish to give up to someone else's care: in effect, she was a victim of her own popularity. Other midwives who had large caseloads did not view it from such a philanthropic point of view, especially as the Medical Officer of Health's attempts to recruit more district midwives were fruitless.

WORKLOAD

Workload was the extent of the midwife's daily duties. These included:

- labour calls/deliveries;
- labour calls/false alarms;
- booking clinics;
- home assessment and advisory visits for all home bookings;
- midwives' antenatal clinics;
- local authority antenatal clinics
- GP antenatal clinics;
- antenatal visits to the home;
- postnatal visits to the home;
- early discharges from hospital-antenatal assessment and visiting postnatally;
- social emergency assessments;
- collecting, checking and recording drugs and arranging destruction of out-of-date drugs;
- collecting and returning equipment;
- sterilizing instruments;
- taking oxygen and gas and air machine for regular checks;
- ensuring car/bicycle maintenance;
- liaison visits with GP, health visitors, social workers, the housing department and the police;

- attending all unbooked and hospital-booked women who gave birth at home;
- attending abortions at home and nursing such women;
- giving cover to her partner/s clients in their absence;
- attending occasional lectures at the health department;
- approved teaching midwives had responsibility for a pupil and/or medical student and/or student nurse.

The workload was related to the number of births and emergencies occurring at any time, thus there were peaks and troughs. Based on an assumption of 100 births per annum and an even work spread, the following is an example of the weekly workload of one district midwife, compiled from information in City of Nottingham MOH report 1961 and midwives' work diaries and oral evidence:

Table 1.1 Estimated weekly workload for one district midwife (home bookings) in 1961

Task	Time
Labour and delivery × 2	13.00
Postnatal visits × 24 estimated visiting time plus travel 45 mins	18.00
Antenatal visits × 12 estimated visiting time plus travel 30 mins	6.00
Special visits × 4 estimated per visit and report 45 mins	3.00
Assessment for social emergency bed × 1 and report	1.00
Midwives booking and antenatal clinic × 1 session	4.00
Parenthood sessions × 1	2.00
Telephone time and record keeping	3.00
Sterilizing equipment, cleaning bags and equipment, washing aprons and uniforms	1.00
Collecting drugs and equipment, visiting health department, attending lectures	1.00
Daily liaison with partner	2.50
Liaison with colleagues, GP, health visitor, social worker, etc.	2.00
Total hours	56.50

Compiled from personal knowledge, oral evidence, City of Nottingham Medical Officer of Health Reports and district midwives' registers and diaries.

In addition to their workload, district midwives were 'on call' for 130 hours in some weeks and less in others (City of Nottingham 1960: 28). At Appendix A *City of Nottingham Health Services Instructions to Midwives* (1957), the reader will get a clear insight into the daily duties of the district midwife, and will see that the time allocated to the tasks above is probably a conservative estimate. This information relates only to workload for home delivery. In addition, city midwives had an ever increasing number of hospital-delivered early discharges for nursing at home, which it is not possible to estimate in terms of cases and time. In reality, the work spread, as in all maternity care, was uneven, resulting in weeks in which the midwives worked for 80 or 90 hours on home-booked cases, and others when they were less busy. The following is one extreme example from a midwife's register of the number of labour calls she attended in one week in 1958:

Table 1.2 Example of deliveries attended by one midwife in one week: March 1958

Date		Time of birth
Sunday	2.5.58	00.15 hrs
Sunday	2.3.58	10.15
Monday	3.3.58	04.30
Tuesday	4.3.58	13.25
Tuesday	4.3.58	21.00
Wednesday	5.3.58	03.45
Thursday	6.3.58	07.20
Friday	7.3.58	02.37

Source: Personal register of a district midwife.

In addition to the births, she would undertake her routine duties; her partner had three deliveries in that week. District midwives' registers indicate that midwives spent an average of 6.50 hours at each delivery; thus in addition to being called out every night this midwife worked in excess of 80 hours in the week in question. The extent of district midwives' daily work routine and professional responsibilities can be seen in the 1957 *Instructions to Midwives*, reproduced at Appendix A.

Olga had this to say:

> I think I held the record for the largest number of deliveries in 48 hours ... I did 7 ... I did a number of 5 in 48 hours, but 7 was the greatest. They are from number 248 in my registers.

Another way of conceptualizing the extent of a district midwife's workload and the variation between individual midwives is shown below. The information is drawn from the personal registers of six city midwives. The number of deliveries relates to workload and not caseload, records annotated* denote that the midwife did not complete a full year's work. This may have been because she began or ended service in that year, had sick leave in excess of one month, a career break or undertook further training. In one instance the missing information is due to lost registers.

The registers were selected to give an example across the time of the study, and to include some period when the six midwives were practising concurrently so that comparative workloads and changes over time can be seen. This example does not show the midwives who on average had the smallest workload or those known to have the largest. It is not intended to imply any statistical significance but merely to show the variation in annual deliveries between midwives in the same domiciliary service, and the shift in the numbers of annual deliveries per midwife over time.

Table 1.3 Six city midwives by number of deliveries per annum: 1951–72

Year	Midwife 1	Midwife 2	Midwife 3	Midwife 4	Midwife 5	Midwife 6
1951	31*	76*				
1952	84	79				
1953	74	96				
1954	72	100				
1955	62	92				
1956	70	105				
1957	55*	114	–	–	133	–
1958	–	–	–	124	109	–
1959	–	–	92	100	89	–
1960	–	–	83	91	63	–
1961	–	–	79	84	76	–
1962	–	107	88	86	69	95
1963	–	110	51*	79	39*	77
1964	79	84	104	66	45	93
1965	70	75	78	68	52	68
1966	71	100	78	53	42	78
1967	61	80	77	62	50	61
1968	84	91	68	45	47	47*
1969	40*	74	71	41	49	62
1970	61	57	57	39	50	62
1971	63	51	65	38	–	64
1972	42	42	40	25	–	33

Source: Personal registers of six district midwives.
*Denotes that the midwife worked only part of the year.

This chart indicates the wide variation in annual deliveries between midwives working full-time in the same domiciliary service. In some instances there are reasons for this. However, it is evident that in most years there was a significant variation in deliveries between midwives, some undertaking twice as many as others: for example, midwife 3 under-took 104 deliveries in 1964, while midwife 5 carried out 45. The number of deliveries undertaken by a midwife in a year had a profound effect upon her workload, as described on pages 9–10 or preceding pages. Women frequently asked midwives who had delivered them but who were not their booked midwife to care for them postnatally. Where this did not require the midwife to travel outside her area, she would usually oblige. Every birth she attended required an average attendance, travel and record-keeping time of approximately ten hours and postnatal visits. In addition, increased deliveries increased the chance of a night call.

Undoubtedly midwives who undertook the most deliveries had the biggest workloads and hours of service.

Interestingly, district midwives did not know how many births their colleagues undertook. The Supervisor of Midwives kept a central record from the birth notifications and each midwife knew how many deliveries she had entered in her register each year, but this information was not published or shared. Supervisors were concerned about the uneven spread of work and tried to address it by asking midwives to keep a district register of all women booked by them for home birth to compare with the number they subsequently delivered. If there was a clear imbalance of bookings and deliveries, the Supervisor would redefine geographical boundaries from time to time to redress that balance. However, while midwife 2 had a relatively high number of births through-out, midwives 4 and 5 began with high returns in the late 1950s and reached a position in 1966 where their average annual births were less than 50% of midwife two. Although the average across the service was still far in excess of the government recommended caseload of 55 per annum, by 1966 midwives 4 and 5 had achieved that target. However, by that time all district midwives were carrying a caseload of women booked for early discharge from hospital following hospital birth. These hospital caseloads quickly exceeded the home-booked caseloads and continued to give district midwives unacceptably high workloads.

The Ministry of Health had expressed concern in 1960 about the working conditions and hours of work of district midwives and asked Medical Officers of Health to publish relief arrangements to ensure that sufficient help was available to cover off duty:

RELIEF ARRANGEMENTS

Owing to the arduous nature of the midwife's work, the Ministry of Health has requested Local Authorities to give details of the arrange-ments in operation for relief duty. The domiciliary midwives work in pairs, relieving each other as far as possible for off duty, holidays and sick leave. The off duty consists of 38 hours for three weekends out of four, an 18 hour period at 2 week-ends and 110 hours at the fourth week-end, allowing five consecutive nights off duty.

(City of Nottingham 1960)

In reality this information was misleading. Most of the midwives worked all week-end, most week-ends. Those given 38 hours off finished 'on call' duty at 8 am on Saturday morning and came back on duty on Sunday evening. If they had been out all night on Friday, they would spend Saturday sleeping. Those given 18 hours off were merely relieved of 'on call' on one night. Those given 110 hours off had their aggregated off duty from previous weeks.

In other words district midwives' working lives included 24 hours of every day. How else could an employer claim to give 'off duty' which merely amounted to one night 'off call', but required full working duties on both days?

Olga recalled something of the good times:

Looking through my registers again, brought back lots of memories, my very first delivery on the district was Mrs … Nottingham's ice-cream family. I was collected from my house by Mr … in his ice-cream van with its ding-dong going (in the early hours) … nothing to hold on to! … when we got to the Bulwell level crossing the gates were down, causing Mr … more panic.

and the bad:

The Winter of 62/63 was unbelievable, delivering babies in the terrible cold weather, if I didn't put the baby straight between the mother's bare breasts, when I got back the baby would be suffering from hypothermia. We often went out in 20° of frost, my buttons used to freeze on my coat and my eye-lashes used to freeze together. I only had an NSU Quickly moped to get about on. I can remember clocking up 100 miles a day.

Because of inadequate cover, midwives frequently struggled to continue working when they were sick or overtired. They knew that there was no one to relieve them in their absence. One retired district midwife made the following statement:

Some of the midwives took drugs from time to time. You have to remember that taking Valium was a way of life for many, GPs prescribed it freely, no one had decided it was dangerous then. GPs surgeries were overflowing with free samples from drugs firms, and they gave them to us for the asking. They knew how tired and over-worked many midwives were. Some of us had spent 20 years being on call every night … out most nights and the continual broken sleep meant we lost the habit of regular sleep. Some midwives took distalgesic or amphetamines … you have to remember that taking these drugs was not seen in the same way then as it is now, half the population was on something.

One of the city mothers in Newson and Newson's 1963 study had this to say about her labour at home:

Oh it was fine … but we had to keep waking the midwife up with cups of tea … it was her fifth in forty eight hours.

(Newson and Newson 1963: 19)

Nevertheless, the city midwives continued to do the best they could for the women of Nottingham. Nellie also recalled the winter of 1962:

> Many of them did a lot of work over and above what was expected ... in spite of the high workload ... a lot of patients got their pipes frozen ... and had no water ... so even if they had washing machines they couldn't use them ... some of the midwives took nappies home and washed and returned them.

In the early 1960s the plight of Nottingham district midwives was made public on a number of occasions through the television, radio and local evening paper:

MIDWIVES REGISTER A PROTEST

Nottingham's midwives spoke out last night about their long hours; of many having a caseload of over 100 confinements a year; and about being taken for granted by the public.

One young woman who recently gave up the profession but has remained in nursing, said: 'I gave it up because of the bad conditions. I had to. My health would not stand those hours. You are on call six days a week – that would not be so bad but often you have to work on right through the night. And you still have to be on duty again the next day.'

This nurse who has been a midwife for six years, had a caseload of over 100. Ideally this should be about 55. But another midwife who regularly tops over 100 in a year has dealt with 44 cases in the last three months. They are concerned about the continued staff shortage which, following a number of staff resignations, is reaching crisis point.

(Nottingham Evening News 2.12.1964)

A further local newspaper report is reproduced on page 15, which elaborates the extent of the arduous life that district midwives were enduring due to the shortage of midwives. When Audrey was asked, in 1991, about her reflections of working conditions during her 20 years on the district, after a few seconds thought she said: 'every night ... when I go to bed I look out of the window before I put the light out, and say, "God bless the night rota" – even now.'

The figures in Table 1.4 (p. 16) include all the midwives who began and ended service on the district and in hospital in any year. They do not represent the average complement of midwives at any time. However, it does indicate the number of district midwives and hospital midwives who gave their intention to practise, by home confinements and hospital deliveries. It also shows the number of midwives working privately or in nursing homes or institutions and latterly those who worked as agency midwives.

go in
pital

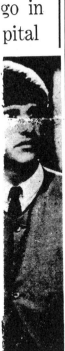

URGENT NEED OF CITY MIDWIVES

CONCERN OVER SHORTAGE

NOTTINGHAM'S overworked midwives are concerned about continued staf
shortages in the city. They feel that the position is reaching crisis poin
following a number of resignations.

Each midwife ideally should deal with a case load of 55 confinements a year but staff shortages and an increasing birthrate means that many of them are coping with double that number.

The Post and News was told today that there were at least three midwife houses standing empty in the city at the moment because of the staffing position.

" Desperate "

There is also a shortage of health visitors in the city—mainly because the working conditions dd not compare favourably with other local authorities.

Nottingham does not pay its health visitors a car allowance. But they have only to cross the river to West Bridgford to work in the county and the allowance is paid.

Some city midwives who have resigned have been refused permission to work part-time, despite the desperate position of the overworked midwives.

Shortage

A spokesman for the Corporation's Health Department today admitted that there was a shortage of midwives and health visitors but denied that the situation had reached crisis proportions.

At present the city had about 44 midwives on its strength—one or two fewer than a year ago.

The birthrate this year was about the same as for 1963.

" I would not say that the situation is any worse now than a year ago," he commented. " Things can change quite quickly. In a month's time we might have a few more midwives back again which could completely change the picture."

Over 3,000 cases

Last year, the city's midwives attended 3,173 confinements — just over half the total births to city mothers.

In addition, many mothers are discharged early from hospital into the care of the city midwifery service.

The increasing birthrate in recent years has also aggravated the position.

Nottingham's hospitals are also trying to recruit more midwives. A drive earlier this year to attract married midwives back into the service resulted in less than a dozen new appointments.

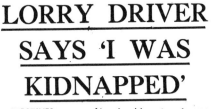

LORRY DRIVER SAYS 'I WAS KIDNAPPED'

DETECTIVES were making inquiries at a transpor
cafe near Grantham today into the alleger
kidnapping of a London lorry driver who was taking
£10,000 worth of shoes to Yorkshire.

The cafe, known as Tony's, is three miles from Grantham on the A1, near Gonerby Moor.

The proprietor told a reporter he could make no comment on the alleged kidnapping.

Meanwhile, police throughout East London started an intensive investigation following the theft of the lorry.

Mr. Albert Fillis (57), of Eltham-road, Eltham, was earlier found on waste ground in Priory-road, Upton Park, London, with a sack tied over his head and arms.

Bulk load

Mr. Fillis, a driver employed by Dolcis Ltd. at their Bermondsey depot, told police that he left the depot for Yorkshire, with a bulk load of shoes, early yesterday.

He said that when he returned to his lorry after a cup of tea at the cafe near Grantham, he was kidnapped, had a sack thrown over his head, and was driven about in the back of the lorry before being dumped in Priory-road.

He was not hurt and a police search found his lorry abandoned near West Ham football ground. The load of shoes was missing.

Stolen in Lincolnshire ?

Grantham CID are investigating reports that the shoes were stolen from the cafe car park.

The cafe, which stays open all night, is at the north end of the Grantham by-pass, and is a favourite stopping place for long-distance lorry men.

'Baby-saver' on the way

A SMALL " kiss of life " pump invented by a Johannesburg doctor to save babies' lives, is to be mass-produced in Britain and the United States because of its remarkable success in South African teaching hospitals.

The resuscitator, claimed to be the first harmless method of inflating a new-born baby's lungs, has a simple mouthpiece that fits over the baby's face and a small hand-operated rubber pump, the air pressure from which is controlled by a valve.

It was originally made by the doctor, an anaesthetist. in his spare time in a home workshop, and can be used by an untrained person.

" Since the new device is nearly foolproof it also ensures the baby does not suffer from a temporary lack of oxygen, which could cause permanent brain damage," said a Johannesburg doctor. " When resuscitating a new-born baby, one is fighting not only for the child's life but for its very wits."

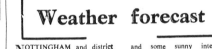

Weather forecast

NOTTINGHAM and district for 24 hours starting noon today, as supplied by the Watnall Meteorological Station. The complex low-pressure

and some sunny intervals. Maximum temperature 41 F, minimum 28 F. Winds variable, becoming north-easterly. light.

Figure 1.2 A local newspaper report reflecting the severe shortage of midwives (1964).

Table 1.4 Midwives giving intention to practise in City of Nottingham

Year	Total home births	Dist. m/ws Prem. m/wvs Supervisors	Hospital births	Hospital m/wvs	Private m/wvs and institutes	Agency mid-wives
1950	2588	37	2538	70	15	0
1955	2521	45	2515	90	17	0
1960	2876	49	2968	76	9	0
1965	2596	49 includes PTS	3548	81	0	0
1970	1404	39 includes PTS	3690	114	0	0
1973	ND	ND	ND	ND	0	24

Source: Medical Officer of Health Reports City of Nottingham.
PTS = part-time staff
ND = no data

These data demonstrate that district midwives delivered on average twice as many babies per annum per midwife as did hospital midwives, despite the fact that they had no support staff and were giving total care to the home-delivered women and postnatal care to those women transferred early from hospital. Except for the occasional presence of a pupil, GP or medical student, they delivered babies single-handedly; indeed 12 of the 14 midwives in the study said that with the exception of the Supervisor of Midwives they had never had another midwife present at a birth.

However, the hospital services were stretched to capacity, every bed was fully booked and constantly occupied. Hospital midwives worked a 42-hour week, but for many the line between work and leisure was often blurred. In order to maintain effective institutional services, staff had to be on duty around the clock. To achieve this across four hospitals required the frequent use of the 'split shift'. On a split shift, the midwife came on duty at 7 am and worked until 12.30 pm, had the afternoon off and returned to work from 5 pm until 9 pm. In reality, the working conditions of hospital midwives, although different, were as unacceptable by today's standards as those of the district midwives.

The number of hospital births rose, although there was an overall fall in total births. Early discharges with transfer of care to district midwives became the norm. By the late 1960s, several district midwives were employed on a part-time basis. The number indicated in Table 1.4 therefore no longer represents only whole-time equivalents after 1965. The part-time midwives were employed to provide relief cover and assistance with postnatal care of hospital-delivered women. However, the repetitious nature of these duties, together with the lack of opportunity for the part-time midwives to utilize their full range of skills was later to lead to a review by the Supervisor of Midwives who decided that all midwives, whether part-time or full-time, should carry a caseload.

MIDWIVES' BOOKING CLINICS AND ANTENATAL CARE

Midwives booking clinics were established at eight centres across the City of Nottingham by 1960. Previously, district midwives had booked women and carried out antenatal care in her own or the mother's home (see illustration on page 18). By 1962 these clinics were well-established in accessible points across the city. During 1962 there were 454 midwives clinic sessions with 11 490 attendances. District midwives also carried out 19 209 antenatal home visits. This set the pattern for the 1960s: by 1967 the balance had changed slightly with 14 116 attendances at midwives clinics and 16 420 home antenatal visits (see illustration on page 18).

TRANSPORT

In the early period of the study, city midwives mostly made their visits on a bicycle. A few who worked in the inner-city area had such small patches, because of the huge number of childbearing women squashed into overcrowded housing, that they were not even eligible for a district bicycle. They carried their equipment from house to house. In 1960 district midwife's equipment was audited by the MOH and found to weigh four stones (City of Nottingham 1960).

Olga gave this recollection from the early 1960s:

> My relief midwife in Mapperley was Mrs ... and as for the first year I only had a push-bike and had trouble keeping the gas and air on the back ... it was very hilly in Mapperley. We arranged that she would put the gas and air down her garden at the side of her loo ... you can imagine the scrambling about that went on in the middle of the night down her garden.

A retired district midwife from a middle-class family background, who at that time was allowed no form of transport, gave this insight into life as a district midwife in the most deprived area of Nottingham in 1947:

> You ran from house to house like a skivvy carrying buckets of boiling water in which you had dropped your instruments from the previous confinement ... I wonder why people wonder what midwives wanted all that boiled water for ... Whilst I loved my profession and the families loved us because they relied on us we were little better off than Victorian housemaids. My family thought

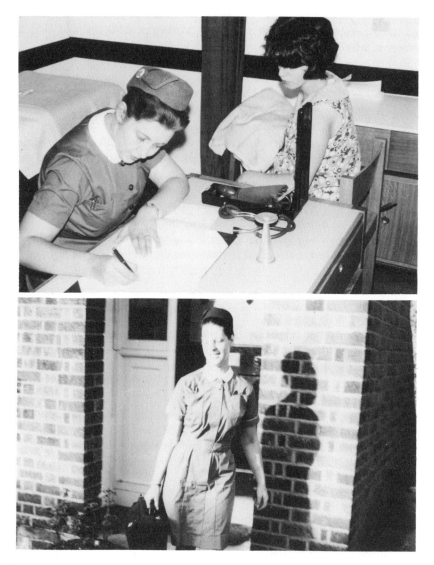

(a)

(b)

Figure 1.3 Antenatal care by the District Midwife (late 1960s). (a) At the clinic. (b) In the home.

> I was crazy for choosing such a job ... they went to no end of trouble to avoid telling people what I did for a living.

Several midwives told me about Miss Millbank (name changed to preserve anonymity):

> Miss Millbank was a popular Nottingham midwife who in the later years of her service began to go blind with cataracts. In those days

midwives did not get their pension unless they completed service to retirement age and Miss Millbank battled bravely on until she was too blind to ride her bike. Eventually it was discovered by her supervisor that she was attending her calls and delivering babies by pushing all her equipment from house to house in an old pram, given to her by one of the mothers. So great was the mothers' loyalty to her that nobody had complained. Finally she was retired from service a few weeks before her official retirement age. After a lot of fuss and threats to expose the Local Authority's meanness to the press she was finally paid her superannuation and pension.

UNIFORMS

While district midwives in many areas wore the national midwives' uniform of stewart blue and grey, some local authorities preferred their midwives' uniforms to be distinctive. The county of Nottinghamshire midwives wore the national uniform but the City of Nottingham district midwives wore green. While most remembered their quality and distinctiveness, there were some mixed feelings. Joyce recalls:

> Green uniforms were because we were 'corporation' midwives, all corporation employees wore green, bus drivers etc. I think it was something to do with Robin Hood.
>
> In the late 1940s and early 1950s our coats were made by Mr Chalk (tailor) on Mansfield Road. Midwives had to go to him to be measured and have a properly tailored coat. We were given a length of green gingham to take to a dressmaker of our choice (for dresses) ... the bill was sent to the Health Department. A man came to the Health Department, from Danco, with a selection of felt and gabardine hats which midwives chose from. There were storm hats, brimmed hats like bowlers, fedoras and winged affairs like air hostesses hats. (See illustration page 20.)
>
> Later all the uniform was supplied by Danco, all made to measure and sent to us individually in a dressmaker's box lined and interleaved with tissue paper. The uniforms were a joy to wear, perfectly fitting and smart.

Audrey so preferred the green local authority uniforms to the navy blue which were issued after the reorganization that she continued to wear green until her retirement in the 1980s. She maintained a supply by collecting the green uniforms of midwives who were handing them in for the new issue. Several attempts were made to encourage her into the new uniform, but none was successful.

Another midwife had this to say:

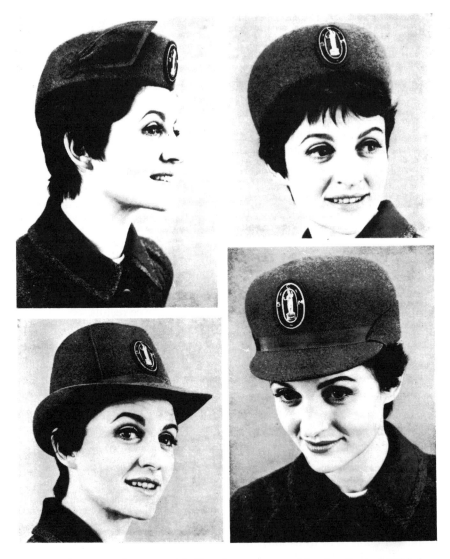

Figure 1.4 1968: The new midwifery hats, approved by the Central Midwives Board.

'We looked like city bus conductresses, all in green, people used to try and give you their fare if you travelled on the bus.'

DRUGS AND INHALATION ANALGESIA

1950 was the first year in which all district midwives were qualified to administer gas and air and the year in which the Dangerous Drugs Regulations authorized midwives to administer pethidine (City of Nottingham 1950/37):

> Regular instruction in the use of gas and air was given to women at antenatal clinics and midwives were trained in the technique of simple relaxation to teach at welfare centres.
>
> *(MOH Report 1951/15)*

The registers contain comprehensive data on drugs, both maternal and paediatric, that district midwives used in labour, at birth and in the immediate postnatal period. Together with the midwives' drugs books, which all the midwives were able to produce, they make the basis of a separate study and no doubt in the fullness of time will be published.

Appendix A (pages 137–138) gives a list of drugs and dosages which were available for use by Nottingham's district midwives in 1957, and gives an idea of the range and complexity of drugs available to district midwives.

WORKING WITH GENERAL PRACTITIONER OBSTETRICIANS

By the 1970s about 80% of Nottingham's GPs were offering maternity medical services (the GPOs). Pregnant women on the list of GPs who did not undertake obstetric care were required to attend another GP for maternity care, while remaining with their own GP for medical care. In terms of continuity of carer this was by no means a satisfactory arrangement.

Some GPOs saw women antenatally during surgery time; others held antenatal clinics. In 1953 one GPO invited a midwife to attend his antenatal clinic (City of Nottingham 1953: 24). In his report in 1958 the Medical Officer of Health had this to say:

> An arrangement from which any benefit to the service is not yet really apparent is the attendance of midwives of some districts at a regular ante-natal session held at general practitioner's surgeries.
>
> *(City of Nottingham 1958: 9)*

By 1969 district midwives were assisting at three GPO antenatal clinics; most resisted attending and several reasons have been cited in oral evidence:

- Midwives resented 'assisting' GPOs (City of Nottingham 1954 and 1969). They considered their normal midwifery skills as equal to those of the GPO, and wished to be considered as partners in the care of childbearing women.
- In their own clinics, midwives often had clinic nurses to assist with weighing, urine testing and blood pressures. They considered that being isolated in a clinical room and given these same tasks by the GPOs reduced their status to that of clinic nurse.

- They seldom saw their own booked clients, as GPs had a wider catchment area than the midwife's geographical patch. This spoilt continuity for some women who saw their own midwife at home and another at the GPO clinic.
- District midwives could not afford the time to attend these clinics.
- Midwives felt that what had been described as an exercise to improve liaison between carers and continuity for clients was wasted, as most of the GPOs never attended home births. (Allison 1991: 39–43).

However, there were some GPOs who took a great interest in the whole childbearing episode, including attendance at delivery. One such GP, who had been senior obstetric registrar for many years, died recently. When interviewed she said that she saw domiciliary midwifery as a happy and safe alternative for women. Of the small percentage of occasions when a GP was called to a home delivery, her name appears the most frequently in the midwives' registers. She would respond to a call for assistance from any district midwife and attend any mother whether or not she was her patient. She expressed the view that if a midwife needed assistance there was frequently nothing a GPO could do that the midwife couldn't. However she chose to attend the births because of her wide obstetric experience, knowing that there was no hope of admitting most women to hospital. In the absence of the opportunity to admit a woman who needed obstetric assistance she felt confident to undertake forceps lift-outs at home.

Sometimes midwives had different experiences, however. Interleaved in the register of one of the midwives was a file note regarding a birth she had attended:

> I asked the husband to call Dr … (GP), but he was put through to the emergency service … meanwhile I had delivered the baby (a brow presentation) … I had done an episiotomy … so I asked the husband to telephone … this time he was given the doctor's number … he came back and said doctor says will you take her to the City hospital … I have no sutures.

Many of the GPOs visited the woman at home after the birth and occasionally during the postnatal period. Apart from the six-week check, all clinical postnatal care for the normal puerperium and normal neonate was carried out by the district midwife. Care of low birthweight babies at home was undertaken by the premature baby midwives.

INTRAPARTUM CARE

The following table illustrates the rise over time in the percentage of women who booked with a GPO for maternity medical services and the fall in the percentage of GPO attendance at birth.

Table 1.5 GPO attendance at home birth: 1951–70

Year	Total home births	Number booked GP	Percentage total births	GP present at birth	Percentage total births
1951	2493	809	32.8	331	13.2
1956	2646	1705	64.4	292	11.0
1960	2876	2237	77.7	214	7.4
1966	2497	2423	96.9	153	6.3
1970	1405	1378	98.0	65	4.6

Source: Medical Officer of Health Reports City of Nottingham 1951–70.
The Medical Officer of Health collated his finding from GP returns. They are at variance with the data in the midwives' birth registers which shows them to have attended births less frequently.

Historically, women visited the district midwife at her home or clinic to book for delivery at home. The view that women voluntarily flocked to the general practitioners after maternity medical care became free within the NHS is not entirely upheld by this study. The fact that the number of women seeking such care increased year on year may have had as much to do with health department directives to midwives to ensure that women attended their GP or welfare clinic as it did with women's desire to seek medical aid (see Appendix A, paragraph 7: Booking).

GPOs indicated if they wished to be present at a birth. In the early days they expected to be informed when labour commenced, and at the beginning of the second stage of labour, or if perineal suturing was required. Towards the end of the period most no longer wished to be informed about labour or to be present at the birth, but simply to be told at the next surgery time when a birth had taken place. Written and oral evidence indicates that the majority of GPOs rarely attended births unless called in an emergency, while a small number of experienced GPOs attended the majority of births where a doctor was present. In 1963, of the 3173 city home births, 3172 were conducted by a district midwife and one by a doctor alone (City of Nottingham 1962: 28).

MATERNITY NURSES

Maternity nursing had previously been defined as: attendance on a woman in childbirth, under the direction and personal supervision of a registered medical practitioner who has been engaged to deliver the patient, has been notified of the onset of labour and remains responsible for the case throughout the lying-in period (Carter and Dodds 1953: 613).

After the implementation of the NHS, the proper role of the midwife in the event of women booking with a general practitioner for maternity care caused some confusion. This was clarified in a circular issued by the Minister of Health in November 1948. Medical practitioners and midwives were informed that, unless a doctor stated specifically that he wished to be summoned at the onset of labour and that he proposed to deliver the woman himself, the midwife was acting as a midwife and not a maternity nurse. With a view to clarifying the matter, a form was issued to medical practitioners to inform the midwife if he had undertaken to provide maternity medical services in a particular case. It also advised her as to whether he did, or did not, wish to be present at the delivery. The form also provided for the midwife to notify the doctor of the result of the delivery if he was not present.

In the event, it quickly became evident that only a minority of general practitioners were interested in intrapartum care and that minority diminished over time. (The level of involvement of GPs can be seen in Table 1.5, p. 23.) The role of and term maternity nurse was abolished in July 1960 (Mason 1963: 13).

LOCAL AUTHORITY ANTENATAL CLINICS

Following the implementation of the NHS, local authority antenatal clinics attended by medical officers continued to function. Some women attended these clinics in addition to seeing their GP and midwife, although on many occasions the district midwife was the only carer present. The number of attendances diminished over time, until they were phased out in the late 1960s.

DISTRICT MIDWIVES AND OBSTETRICIANS

Obstetricians played no part in the care of most women booked for home birth in Nottingham; more than 95% of women delivered at home neither visited the maternity hospital nor saw an obstetrician. Due to the maternity-bed shortage in Nottingham, no woman booked for home birth would be referred to or booked with an obstetrician except in an obstetric or social emergency. However, there was a supportive relationship between district midwives and obstetricians in Nottingham. Under an arrangement with the obstetricians, midwives were able to transfer women to hospital in labour or emergency and to call for the flying squad without prior consultation with a GP. On occasions, obstetricians visited women 'on the district', and occasionally performed procedures at home following a request for an opinion from a GP or midwife. Sometimes an obstetrician would perform inductions at home to avoid admissions to the overcrowded maternity hospital.

Olga recalls: 'Mr ... (obstetrician) came round with me one Thursday with his Drew Smythe catheter ... inducing the overdue women ... this made sure that I had a very busy weekend'. For a number of years there was also a small peripheral obstetric clinic where GPs or midwives could refer women for an opinion. It was phased out, apparently through lack of use.

DISTRICT TRAINING OF PUPIL MIDWIVES: CITY OF NOTTINGHAM

Pupils from the local Part 2 training school spent a minimum of three months with a city midwife. In the early post-war years they lived with their teaching midwife, working six days and on call six nights a week. Many of the midwives had interesting stories to tell about their district training. This is Joyce's story about her district midwifery training during the war:

> You worked, ate and spent your recreation time alongside her (teaching district midwife) ... Since you were always on call, night and day, it wasn't possible, even, to go out for a walk alone ... in the evening. My district midwife was a middle aged single lady ... on her day off I was expected to visit her mother with her. In the evenings we sat together ... I found this very difficult to accept, by nature I'm a solitary person ... I like to read ... prefer my own company. ... There was no recognition of the fact that I was an individual, a young woman in my middle twenties ... why did we accept this and didn't complain ... it never occurred to us to complain, to go against the system ... it would have been received with incredulity, we would have been considered very ungrateful and disruptive. ... My midwife wasn't unkind ... she felt that she was doing me a kindness ... including me in her life, but I was never asked how I felt about it. She did allow my boyfriend ... [the man she later married] to visit me ... in the evenings.

This is Annie's story about life as a district pupil in the 1940s:

> I lived with a district midwife whose mother was an undertaker ... she dressed all in black ... long clothes ... like Queen Mary. The coffins were made in her front room ... and stored there ... up against the walls. Well ... I had to keep my bicycle in there amongst the coffins. If I got called out in the night ... I had to creep in there

C.M.B. Rules Without Tears: 3

A light-hearted pictorial guide to some of the rules of the Central Midwives Board, by Miss G. L. Reed, S.C.M., S.R.N., R.F.N., Midwifery Tutor, St. Mary's Hospitals, Manchester

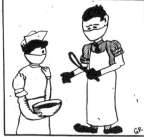

RULE E 12, In all cases of illness of the patient or child, or of any abnormalities occurring during pregnancy, labour or lying-in, a midwife must call to her aid a registered medical practitioner

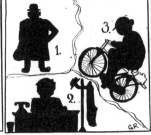

RULE E 14, The midwife must notify the Local Supervising Authority whenever medical aid has been sought, give a copy to the doctor and retain one for herself

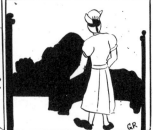

RULE E 15, Whenever a doctor has been sent for, the midwife obtains instructions from him and must obey them. When danger is threatened await arrival of doctor. If doctor is not available in emergency the midwife must remain and do her best until emergency is over

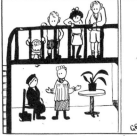

RULE E 16 (a, b, and c), When engaged to attend a patient, the midwife must interview, inquire and advise on ante-natal care and must see patient during pregnancy as often as is necessary

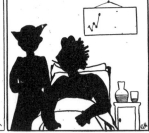

RULE 18, The midwife must take and record accurately the pulse-rate and temperature of the patient at each visit, recording dates and times in a note-book or chart, carefully preserved

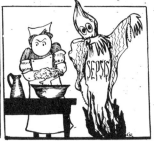

RULE E 20, The midwife must not make more internal examinations than are absolutely necessary

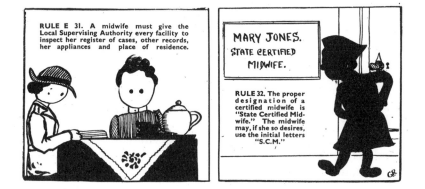

RULE E 31. A midwife must give the Local Supervising Authority every facility to inspect her register of cases, other records, her appliances and place of residence.

MARY JONES.
STATE CERTIFIED MIDWIFE.

RULE 32. The proper designation of a certified midwife is "State Certified Midwife." The midwife may, if she so desires, use the initial letters "S.C.M."

Figure 1.5 Cartoons from The Nursing Mirror to aid recall of the Central Midwives Board Rules.

in the dark … find my bicycle and wheel it out … my heart used to pound like a drum … silly really. When she attended a funeral she dressed all in black undertaker's clothes and walked at the head of the procession … sometimes I'd see her when I was out doing calls … when she got back she always said … 'Well I gave him a right good send off'.

The *Nursing Mirror* did attempt to lighten the starchy side of midwifery training for wartime pupils, who were to become the midwives of the new NHS, by publishing a series of cartoons to aid recall of the Central Midwives Board rules (see page 26).

Later, there was a designated hostel where some district midwives and the pupils lived. Until the 1960s, pupils in Nottingham undertook at least 30 home deliveries in their district placement, many unattended by the midwife or general practitioner. Even in the early 1970s they were assured of at least ten home births. District placements helped pupils to consolidate their experience and to prepare to work independently. Undoubtedly this was a key factor in preparing midwives for the type of care they were expected to offer, and in helping them to determine in which setting they preferred to work.

THE TEACHING DISTRICT MIDWIFE: CITY OF NOTTINGHAM

Selected midwives were approved through the local midwifery training school as district teaching midwives and they were guaranteed a continuous stream of pupils. District midwives who took on a teaching responsibility received an additional payment (see pay slip illustration) but were expected to take on more cases as pupils were considered experienced enough to take on some deliveries and routine care on their own by the end of the district placement. These midwives were selected for their high standards of practice and aptitude and commitment to teaching. In 1949 there were nine teaching district midwives in Nottingham; in 1970 there were 12. Between 1949 and 1970, 719 pupil midwives did their district training with this small band of teachers.

DISTRICT TRAINING OF UCH MEDICAL STUDENTS BY NOTTINGHAM'S DISTRICT MIDWIVES

Between the years 1956 and 1966, city midwives supervised the district midwifery training of medical students from University College Hospital, London; 76 medical students attended 345 home births with city midwives (City of Nottingham 1957–66).

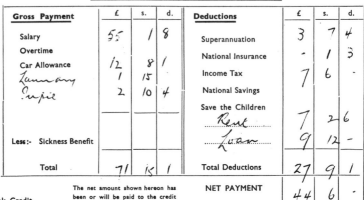

CITY OF NOTTINGHAM.

Statement of Salary Payment for Month ending DEC 1957

Details of Calculation of Net Payment :—

Gross Payment	£	s.	d.	Deductions	£	s.	d.
Salary	55	1	8	Superannuation	3	7	4
Overtime				National Insurance	-	1	3
Car Allowance	12	8	1	Income Tax	7	6	-
Laundry	1	15		National Savings			
Pupil	2	10	4	Save the Children			
				Rent	7	2	6
Less:- Sickness Benefit				*Loan*	9	12	-
Total	71	15	1	Total Deductions	27	9	1

Bank Credit

The net amount shown hereon has been or will be paid to the credit of your personal account not later than the above date.

NET PAYMENT	44	6	-

SALS. P3.

CITY OF NOTTINGHAM.

Statement of Salary Payment for Month ending ....

Details of Calculation of Net Payment :—

Gross Payment	£	s.	d.	Deductions	£	s.	d.
Salary	55	1	8	Superannuation	3	7	4
Overtime				National Insurance		2	1
Car Allowance *Laundry*	25	7	3	Income Tax	8	13	-
Medical Students	5	15	2	National Savings			
				Save the Children			
				Rent	7	2	6
Less:- Sickness Benefit				*Loan*	9	12	-
Total	86	4	1	Total Deductions	28	16	11

Bank Credit

The net amount shown hereon has been or will be paid to the credit of your personal account not later than the above date.

NET PAYMENT	57	7	2

SALS. P3.

Figure 1.6 Two pay slips reflecting the midwives' monthly salary indicating the extra pay for additional responsibilities.

The city midwives took the medical students in their stride and gave them no special treatment. The students were expected to attend the calls in the same capacity as pupil midwives, except that they were never left to undertake the delivery alone. They were required to look after the woman in labour, to assist in preparing the room and to carry out routine observations in labour. Most importantly, they had to make themselves acceptable to the woman and her family at whose discretion they were allowed in the house.

One teaching midwife had this to say:

> They were generally a nice bunch ... eager to learn ... a bit frightened of us ... and very respectful to the families, however poor they were. For a lot of them it was a shock ... during the night hours they would talk about their families ... it was plain that most had never seen this side of life ... only read about it ... I don't remember one that didn't enjoy it or benefit ... one or two needed taking down a peg ... or at least seeing what life was about ... they saw it in Radford ... [inner city area]. I enjoyed having them ... I learned what was going on in hospital.

It was acknowledged by medical educationalists that student doctors had something to learn from district midwives about normal birth which they could not experience anywhere else. The relationship which was forged between medical student, midwife and pupil midwife acted as a foundation for future understanding of the role and interdependence of the two professions.

APPOINTMENT AND GRADE

District midwives were appointed by the Medical Officer of Health; the annual complement varied between 26 and 44 with an average of 33, including the premature baby midwives, who did not undertake deliveries (City of Nottingham 1949–72). They were appointed as midwifery sisters from the first day of service and supported by their partner for a negotiated period. There was a length-of-service related, incremental pay scale, but no midwife held a superior rank to another. There were no team leaders: each midwife was accountable to the Supervisor of Midwives for her practice, and had a duty to remain in communication with her partner to ensure reciprocal cover for their clients.

All written and oral evidence indicates that this system worked well. Indeed, in discussion with the retired midwives every one of them found today's grading of midwives and notion of requiring mentorship after training difficult to comprehend. In conversation, the retired midwives did not see any of today's many concepts of team midwifery as equating to the way in which they worked. They perceived themselves to have been individual practitioners, working with a partner/s for the benefit of the client. They had no understanding of what role a team leader could fulfil; when I suggested a comparison with a GP partnership they felt that this more clearly defined the manner in which domiciliary midwifery was organized.

> M: I don't understand about these leaders ... who do they lead ... do you mean supervisors?
>
> JA: No ... well ... not necessarily ... it would be like the partnership you worked in with Mrs G and Mrs H ... but one of you would be the leader, the boss ... would organize the work ... off duty ... the management of the partnership.
>
> M: We did that for ourselves ... I don't think that would have washed with city midwives ... our boss was the supervisor ... Miss Lambert ... she managed all of us and the prems ... and did clinics ... and paperwork for Dr Dodd [MOH] ... we just did the deliveries ... looked after our patients ... we didn't need a leader.

SUPERVISION OF MIDWIVES

From the oral evidence of the supervisors the following list of duties has been constructed:

- 24-hour cover by one of the two supervisors for emergency contact by district midwives;
- three monthly supervisory visits to midwives' homes for record and drug checks;
- arranging off-duty and 24-hour cover for all labours and emergencies in the City; arranging placements for district pupils, medical students and student nurses;
- holiday rotas;
- issuing prescriptions;
- issuing, replacing, checking uniform and equipment;
- teaching district pupils about maternal and child public health issues 2 x 1 hour per week;
- acting as a relief for clinics when midwives were attending a birth;
- attending births in a supervisory capacity – sometimes with pupils;
- taking parentcraft sessions;
- collecting and collating data for the MOH;
- report writing for the MOH.

This is how Nellie, a retired supervisor, described her day:

> In a day you dealt with midwives coming into the office for prescriptions for Pethidine ... for uniforms ... equipment changing ... we did a lot of paperwork for the MOH ... sorting out the records that were kept. I used to attend clinics and parentcraft ... they were all short of manpower ... the birth-rate was so high ... you couldn't guarantee all the midwives would be there. I kept my hand in at clinical teaching ... I used to take the district pupils twice a week for an hour's tuition ... I took them in a room in the Health Department. I also used to do revision on midwifery aspects as well as the public health side.

The following is one example, from 1955, of the annual workload in terms of supervision, of the supervisors of midwives in the City of Nottingham:

Table 1.6 Work done by the Supervisor of Midwives and Assistant Supervisor City of Nottingham 1955

Visits to midwives and inspection of records and equipment	184
Inspection of midwives in nursing homes	11
Special domiciliary visits:	
Expectant and nursing mothers	229
Stillbirths	10
Puerperal pyrexia	32
Skin conditions	14
Office interviews regarding hospital confinements	571

Source: Medical Officer of Health Report 1955.

The pattern of supervisory duties remained fairly constant until the late 1960s.

SUPERVISORY VISITS TO THE MIDWIFE'S HOME

On the appointed day of a supervisory visit, the midwife had ready her records, registers, casenotes, drug book, drug box, work diary, uniform and equipment and any locally required records. She would need to show evidence of her clinic work, attendances and follow-up. In addition, her equipment was checked and her uniform, bag linings and gowns were also counted and inspected. The place where her drugs were stored in her home was checked for security and any rooms in which she interviewed or examined women were inspected for cleanliness and appropriateness. A supervisory visit would take at least half a day to complete. All records were examined and registers and casenotes were checked against the drug

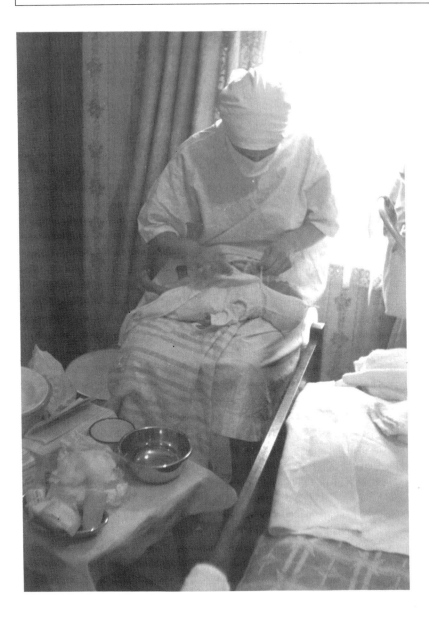

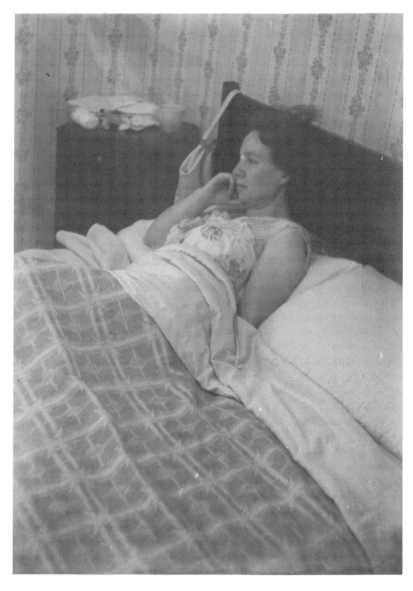

Figure 1.7 Watching the premature baby midwife care for her low birthweight baby, *c.* 1960.

records and prescriptions. Critical incidences, such as stillbirths, maternal deaths and occasions when the flying squad was called would be reflected upon. At the end of the session the supervisor would sign and date the midwives' register in red ink. The registers of the City and County of Nottingham' district midwives demonstrate that this task was assiduously carried out, throughout the years of this study.

PREMATURE BABY MIDWIVES

In 1950 one district midwife undertook the 'Premature Baby Care Course' at the Sorrento Maternity Hospital, Birmingham. From then until the system was disbanded in the 1980s, three or four premature baby midwives were employed to undertake from birth the care of low birth-weight babies born at home. Latterly, they took on the care of small babies transferred from hospital. During the years 1952 to 1966, they cared for 2051 low birthweight babies at home with remarkably good success (details and discussion can be found on page 100).

Where a small or premature baby was anticipated, the premature baby midwife would be informed beforehand but would rarely be present at the birth. The care of mother and baby was shared between district midwife and premature baby midwife to ensure as much continuity and mutual support as possible. The Medical Officer of Health recognized in his 1953 memorandum outlining policy for the care of low birthweight babies that small babies born at home usually 'did better' if they were kept at home. Figure 1.7 shows a Nottingham mother watching the premature baby midwife bath her baby.

MARITAL STATUS OF NOTTINGHAM'S DISTRICT MIDWIVES

A frequently expressed belief is that district midwives were usually single and childless, dedicated to their calling, sacrificing their own chance of family life for the vicarious experience of working with mothers and babies.

In the following table, the number of midwives practising on the district has been taken entirely from the few remaining official lists of city midwives. These were amended and republished several times each year. The lists were distributed by the supervisor to the district midwives, midwives clinics, general practitioners and hospitals. The marital state and whether or not the midwives were mothers was derived from the oral evidence of the supervisor in 1957 and 1969, and my own recollection of the midwives of 1972.

Table 1.7 Marital status of district midwives in Nottingham: 1957, 1969 and 1972

Year	Number of midwives on official list	Marital status: single		Marital status: married		Married midwives with children:	
		number	%	number	%	number	%
1957	33	19	56	14	44	9	64
1969	29	11	38	18	62	15	83
1972	27	10	37	17	63	13	76

Compiled from official lists of city midwives, oral evidence and author's knowledge.

In 1957, 44% of city midwives were married, divorced, separated or widowed, most with children, although the majority of 56% were single. In 1972, 63% were married, divorced, separated or widowed, 76% of whom had children.

Although the position changed over time, it is clear that married women were always a substantial part of the district midwifery workforce in Nottingham. It may be that the greater number of unmarried midwives in the early part of the study had more to do with the death of young men in the war than the self-sacrifice of women to midwifery as a vocation incompatible with family life.

STATUS OF DISTRICT MIDWIVES IN SOCIETY

From interviews with ten retired district midwives, it is clear that they had a sense of their own worth, especially those who worked during Phase One. They saw themselves as individual practitioners working with others to ensure cover for their clients in their absence. They recognized that they had a duty to the public and an accountability to their supervisor.

They gave examples of why they had this sense of 'high professional status':

- high visibility in the community;
- welcome in family homes;
- everybody knew the name of the local midwife and where she lived;
- everybody knew the time and place of the local midwives clinic;
- women came back to them time and again for their services;
- kindnesses shown by poor families;
- asked to be godparents many times;
- recognized by family as 'our midwife';
- high quality, tailormade and distinctive uniforms;
- headed note-paper, with midwife's name, address and telephone number with the local authority logo;

- printed visiting cards;
- designated clinics with secretarial assistance, clinic nurse, and child minding support;
- midwives houses, provided by the local authority;
- house nameplates (state certified midwife);
- City of Nottingham midwife car signs;
- midwife's authority to recommend women for hospital booking;
- midwife's authority to approach social services and housing department;
- midwife's authority to make direct referrals to an obstetrician;
- the respect that obstetricians showed towards district midwives and their midwifery prowess;
- the acknowledgement given to them by the Medical Officer of Health;
- hot meals provided for them at the midwives' hostel every lunch-time by the house-keeper.

Most of the midwives valued the relationships that developed with 'their' families. To be asked to be a godparent was viewed as the ultimate acknowledgement of their acceptability to those families: all had been asked at some time to act as godparent. One midwife had seven godchildren and had been asked on more occasions but had declined after the seventh as she took the role of godmother seriously and felt she could not do justice to any more. Several of the midwives were able to produce photographs of these now grown-up children and two displayed their framed photographs in their living-room.

WORKING IN PARTNERSHIP WITH COLLEAGUES AND FAMILIES

In keeping with contemporary behaviour, district midwives conducted themselves in a more formal manner than today. Two retired midwives recalled that those who were not married frequently lived a solitary single existence either in a nurses' home, hostel or district house. They sometimes shared their life with a female relative or professional colleague, never with a man unless married.

This insular and industrious life was encouraged both by society and the employer. Almost always on call, there was little opportunity for socializing other than at such occasions as were convened at the hospital, hostel or welfare centre where ready access to the midwife could be gained. Similarly, married district midwives would spend almost every evening at home 'on call'.

Even their day-to-day communication with each other and their clients was much more conservative than today. Partners usually addressed each other by their surname: thus my partner was known to me as 'Knight', and I to her as 'Allison'. Whether this trait was peculiar to Nottingham has not been established. Mothers, whatever their social status, would always be addressed as Mrs, even on the rare occasion that their marital status was in doubt. Pupils, whether direct entry or nurse qualified, were addressed by the prefix Nurse, to ensure that any professional with whom they came into contact was aware that they were not yet qualified as a midwife, while mothers and families, however long they had known her, always addressed their midwife either as Miss/Mrs or Nurse, followed by their surname (see letter page 83).

CONCLUSION

An unequivocal finding of this chapter is that domiciliary midwives in Nottingham worked on the district because that is where they choose to be. Many trained with a view to employment in the domiciliary midwifery service and frequently remained there throughout their working life. They had a measure of expertise and autonomy in their chosen field that gave them confidence and arguably inspired confidence in the women for whom they cared. They gave a comprehensive, woman-centred service, guaranteeing continuity of carer and the enormous satisfaction of knowing their value to society.

There is no doubt that their caseloads were too large, unequally distributed and their working hours were difficult. Nevertheless, they remained working 'on the district', when there was ample opportunity to take a hospital midwifery post with regular hours. For those who were nurse trained, the chance of returning to nursing was always there, but the only example of this was the one recorded in the local paper (see page 14).

The 1949 working party (Carter and Dodds 1953) recognized the unique service given by domiciliary midwives and specified that: 'The status of midwives should be safeguarded ... they should be regarded as colleagues of doctors and not merely as maternity nurses working under the orders of a doctor.' This was echoed in all subsequent reports on the maternity services and in Medical Officer of Health reports (City of Nottingham 1949: 36) until 1970, when the Peel Report recommended that: 'Continuity of patient care is best achieved by continuity of association of particular groups of midwives with particular general practices, based where possible in group practices or health centres.'

In 1973 the locally based district midwifery service was disbanded and a cross-functional management system was put in place. District midwives were renamed community midwives and within five years women's choice of a planned birth at home was no longer a reality. In 1980 less than 1% of babies were born at home in Nottingham and the majority of those were not planned to take place there (Allison 1991: 30).

By the late 1970s, NHS employers demanded that midwives had two years' hospital experience before applying for a community post. Midwifery training had been reduced to a single period and direct entry training was being phased out. As the home birth rate reduced, midwives were unable to gain enough district experience to give them the confidence and skills they required. Today many midwives may never have seen a home birth, let alone undertaken one.

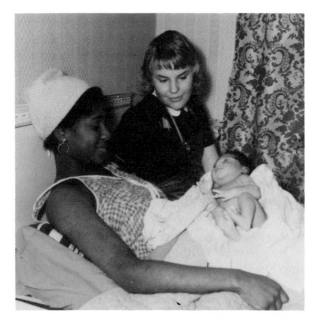

Figure 1.8 The end of an era: district midwife and mother admire her baby shortly after a home birth. Father took the picture, early 1970s.

WORK AND LIFE OF DISTRICT MIDWIVES

Key Points

- District midwifery care was provided by a discrete district-based service, within the wider framework of public health.
- Chief executive officers were required to have a midwifery/maternity service/public health background.
- Health departments were local authority based, unrelated to hospital acute services.
- Supervisors of midwives were clinically linked and district based.
- The majority of direct entrants were employed as district midwives.
- Married women were always a substantial part of Nottingham's district midwifery workforce.
- More direct entrants remained in practice compared to midwives who were registered nurses.
- Between 1947 and 1964 in Nottingham, continuity of carer for women having a home birth was guaranteed.
- In 1949 the recommended annual caseload for an urban district midwife was 55. In 1963 the caseload of district midwives in Nottingham was 106.
- The majority of GPs offered maternity medical services. In 1970 they attended 65 (4.6%) of the 1405 births which occurred at home in Nottingham.
- Pupil midwives usually undertook 30 home births during their district placement.
- District midwives in Nottingham supervised the district midwifery training of 76 medical students from University College Hospital, London.
- District midwives were individual practitioners working in partnerships. No midwife held a superior rank to another and there were no team leaders.
- District midwives believed they had a 'high professional status' in society.

Choosing the place of birth

In the first chapter we looked at how district midwives lived and worked and concluded that their work was in one sense an extension of their life and home. District midwives were almost exclusively employed to deliver women at home, to provide the function of the local authority domiciliary service. However, for the mothers of Nottingham deciding where their baby would be delivered was not simply a matter of informed choice or of fulfilling the criteria for a home birth. In this chapter, issues central to determining where women gave birth in Nottingham during this period are discussed. In consequence, the familiar argument that women who were delivered at home were low risk for complication loses its impact.

In order to put the domiciliary midwifery service into context, an overview of the places of birth and types of maternity carer, including the likelihood of continuity of carer, available to the women of Nottingham are described. Second, the criteria which were applied to women and their circumstances to decide where their baby would be born, and to what extent women in Nottingham fulfilled those criteria, are disclosed. Finally, the extent to which women were selected or able to choose their place of birth or carer is discussed together with the degree of continuity of carer that the various choices offered.

Nottingham lagged behind the rest of the country in moving towards hospitalization of birth due to a shortage of hospital maternity beds. The following is an overview of options for place of birth and/or carer in Nottingham, including the number of births which occurred in the various systems during the period of the study.

There were 76 287 hospital births to City of Nottingham residents between 1948 and 1972. Eighty per cent took place in the maternity wards of the city's general and women's hospitals, and 20% at the only maternity hospital. The vast majority of home births were undertaken by city midwives: between 1948 and 1972 they carried out 62 444 home deliveries.

The number of births occurring in private nursing homes diminished over time: in 1950, 214 were recorded in an unspecified number of homes, while in 1967 the number had reduced to 26 in one (City of Nottingham 1950 and 1967: 29). In addition, the maternity hospital offered amenity beds, which for payment of a fee ensured extra privacy but no priority of care.

Table 2.1 Place and number of births and continuity of carer in Nottingham 1948–1972

Place	Number of births	Annual examples	Number of carers per woman	Chance of known carer at delivery
Choice of four NHS Hospitals	76 287	2538 in 1950 3604 in 1967	1–16	Good
NHS-LA home delivery	62 444	2588 in 1950 2216 in 1967	1–4	Guaranteed
Private nursing home	Data incomplete	214 in 1950 26 in 1967	No data	Probably good
Independent midwives	Data incomplete	20 in 1950 11 in 1962	1	Guaranteed
Independent doctors	Data incomplete	8 in 1949 1 in 1956	No data	No data

Source: Allison 1991, Medical Officer of Health Reports 1949–72 and oral evidence.

The number of home births undertaken by private midwives diminished from 20 births by five midwives during 1950 to 11 births by one midwife in 1962, after which time there were none (City of Nottingham 1950 and 1962: 32). On occasions, home births were undertaken by private doctors: eight occurred in 1949 and one in 1956, after which no more appear to have taken place (City of Nottingham 1949 and 1956). There were no GPO unit facilities in Nottingham during the time of this study.

An interesting feature of this data is the way in which private (independent) practice by both midwives and doctors rapidly disappeared after the introduction of the National Health Service; for midwives it was a trend which had begun with the requirement of the 1936 Midwives Act for Local Supervising Authorities (LSAs) to provide a domiciliary midwifery service.

Oral evidence suggests that the private midwives still practising after the introduction of the NHS had failed to take the opportunity to come into the City's domiciliary service because they could not accept the hours or conditions of service or were near to retirement and happy to end their career looking after a few of the 'regular families' they had served for years. Once a free local authority domiciliary midwifery service became established, with its smartly turned-out midwives who lived in the locality, carrying all the latest equipment and offering continuity of carer the demand for independent midwives disappeared. One of the district midwives who practised during and shortly after the Second World War had this to say about the few 'private' midwives she knew:

> I suppose if I am honest we [district midwives] looked down our noses at them ... it sounds awful to say now but we really thought of them as 'inferior' to us ... they seemed to struggle to get by and they seemed a relic of the past ... not always up to date.

Most of the district midwives I talked to could not remember ever knowing a private midwife. It is worthy of note that the demand for independent practitioners arose again in the 1980s following the demise of a viable home delivery service.

CRITERIA FOR HOME BIRTH

As the case against home birth developed, the number of medical, obstetric and social conditions said to contraindicate home birth grew. Criteria for home birth were published from time to time from the late 1950s (Campbell and Macfarlane 1987). In 1967 the Ministry of Health published in their booklet *Safer Obstetric Care* criteria which should apply at booking for normal (home or GP unit) birth. Although these particular criteria were not developed until 1967, they will be applied as a measure across all the home deliveries in the study in order to demonstrate the percentage of women delivered at home, throughout the period, who by the end of the era were considered 'high risk'.

Ministry of Health Criteria for Normal (Home) Confinement: Booking Arrangements
- As far as can be ascertained the woman's general physical state is unimpaired.
- She is pregnant for the second, third or fourth time, the previous pregnancies, labour and puerperia having been normal and she is under 35 years of age or, if a primipara, she is under 30 years of age.
- She is known to have no Rhesus antibodies.
- The home conditions are suitable.

In relation to the woman's parity, the second criterion is not clear. While stating that the woman, at booking, should be pregnant for the second, third or fourth time the statement is then qualified with the proviso 'if a primipara', she is under 30 years of age. The meaning of primipara is a woman who has given birth to her first child, thus she must be pregnant for at least the second time when booking. There is no reason given why a primipara should be less than 30 years of age. Thus women pregnant for the first time have been counted, and those over 30 years of age are separately identified.

No mention is made of the relationship of fundal height to dates, multiple or young teenage pregnancies. Some of the multiple pregnancies were booked for home birth and others were undiagnosed. However, multiple pregnancy had long been identified as a cause for booking for hospital birth; thus multiple pregnancies have been counted as contraindicating booking for home birth.

On the other hand, the final criterion relates to the suitability of home conditions, and in this regard girls less than 16 years of age, in addition to their obstetric risk, have been counted as unsuitable for home delivery. Such girls were always unmarried, mostly unsupported by the father of the baby, almost always experiencing unplanned pregnancies in the period in question and would have been living with their parents or in the care of the local authority. The majority fell within the 'high risk', unbooked, no antenatal care group.

These criteria apply to a prospective birth, the woman at booking; if judgement is to be made retrospectively about which women fulfilled the criteria for home birth two other elements must be added:

- pregnancies of minimum 36 weeks duration when labour commences;
- pregnancies of maximum 42 weeks duration when labour commences.

Cases which fell outside these parameters were generally accepted to indicate the need for referral or hospitalization (City of Nottingham 1953); thus such births did not fulfil the criteria for a home birth.

TO WHAT EXTENT DID WOMEN IN NOTTINGHAM FULFIL THESE CRITERIA?

Just to sit and peruse the midwives' registers shows the reader that women who gave birth at home at that time had very different obstetric and social backgrounds to those which would be considered appropriate for a home booking today. Evidence of this can be seen on page 97, where from the records of 20 women with multiple pregnancies who were delivered at home, it can be seen that 45% had contraindications to home birth in addition to their multiple pregnancy. Likewise, the extracts from the registers at Appendix C tell an interesting story.

In order to test further the likely extent to which the 62 444 women delivered at home in Nottingham between 1948 and 1972 matched the 1967 Ministry of Health criteria for home birth, the records of the 11 850 home deliveries in this study have been examined. The sample represents 19% of home births in Nottingham in the period, from the registers of 14 midwives. It includes home births from every year between 1948 and 1972 and across the whole area of the city. However, there is no way of proving that this sample is absolutely representative of births across the time frame and geographical boundaries of the study, nor is there a likelihood of increasing the sample. Table 2.2 shows that 6162 (52%) of the 11 850 women delivered at home in this sample did not fulfil the criteria for home birth, for one or more reasons.

Table 2.2 Home deliveries in Nottingham between 1948 and 1972, by reasons why some women, from a sample of 11 850, did not fulfill the 1967 criteria for home birth

Reason	Number out of 11 850 women delivered at home	Percentage
Gestation		
−36 weeks gestation	497	4.20
+42 weeks gestation	1659	14.00
Age, parity, multiparity		
twins/multiple	62	0.52
−16 years	101	0.85
Primigravidae −30	1967	16.60
Primigravidae +30	106	0.90
+35 yrs and known medical conditions	1179	9.95
Total reasons	8466	
Not booked for home delivery	477	4.03
Total women with one or more reason for not fulfilling criteria	6162	52.00

Source: personal registers of 14 City of Nottingham midwives.

Column one lists the causes for falling outside the criteria for home birth. Columns two and three indicate the number and percentage of the 11 850 women in the study who fell outside the criteria for home birth by reason. Some women fell outside the criteria by more than one reason.

There were 8466 known reasons why women in the study did not fulfil the criteria for home birth, although some women had more than one cause, such as the 45-year-old unbooked gravida 17 who had a successful home birth, the many primigravidae, over 30 years of age, who had pregnancies of longer than 42 weeks, and women with multiple pregnancies and other contraindicating factors. In all, 52%, 6162 of women in the sample, did not fulfil the criteria for home birth by one or more factors.

There is no reason to believe that this sample of 19% of home births across the time and spread of district midwives and locations in Nottingham during the period in question does not represent the general picture. 11 850 women, 477 (4.03%) were unbooked for home birth, compared with the 1806 (3.2%) of all women in Nottingham in the same period (page 71) estimated to have been delivered at home though unbooked or hospital booked. This comparison indicates that the estimated figure has not been overstated.

It is evident from this sample that criteria for home birth were much more loosely applied than had previously been assumed. The shortage of hospital maternity beds ensured that the hospitalization of all women who did not fulfil the criteria for home birth was never achieved in Nottingham during the life of the local authority domiciliary midwifery service. This is not to say, however, that no attempts were made to address the issue of ensuring that women perceived to be most in need of hospital birth were ensured a bed.

APPLICATION FOR HOSPITAL BED ON SOCIAL GROUNDS

The condition of post-war housing was a matter of concern throughout the country: war-damaged, old, overcrowded and insanitary housing was badly in need of replacement and repair. The evidence of the MOH Reports, the midwives' registers and the Perinatal Motality Survey 1958 (Butler and Bonham 1963: 289) indicate that despite the provision of hospital maternity beds, the bias to home birth was among those in the poorest conditions. Most district midwives in Nottingham worked primarily with such families. The following extracts from contemporary Medical Officer of Health Reports give insight to the prevailing housing conditions:

> In housing progress was made in the displacement of the occupiers from houses in the Sneinton Elements Clearance Area where one

hundred and five unsatisfactory houses will be demolished as soon as the occupants can be displaced. Emphasis must be given to the fact that the housing position is still a matter of concern ... only those houses that are too dilapidated, insanitary and incapable of repair can be eliminated. In the latter cases not only do the tenants of the houses need rehousing but often sub-tenants and their families also, due to the fact that members of the tenants family have grown up and married and continued to live with parents.

(City of Nottingham 1951)

In addition to slum clearance, councils and corporations across the country were endeavouring to make inroads into the ever-growing list of housing defects. In 1951 Nottingham City Council carried out 10 328 housing repairs ranging from roofs to floors and coppers used to boil the weekly 'whites' wash (City of Nottingham 1951).

The local authority acknowledged the risk to mothers and babies of confinement in unhygienic and overcrowded circumstances by the provision of a quota of hospital beds for social reasons. Using a 'home assessment form', city midwives assessed the homes of those with poor social conditions and made recommendations for hospital beds. The interview, conducted by way of the midwife asking questions and completing a questionnaire, addressed the following issues:

- How many families lived in the house?
- Was there an indoor lavatory?
- How many families shared the lavatory?
- Was there a bathroom?
- How many families shared the bathroom?
- Was there a running water supply inside the house?
- If no indoor running water supply, where was the nearest tap?
- Was there a means of heating water?
- Was there a means of heating the room in which the birth would take place?
- Did the woman and her husband have exclusive use of a bedroom?
- If shared with a child/children, how old were they and could they be put in another room for the delivery?
- How many other children were there in the family relative to the available space and support?
- Did the woman have suitable help for the delivery and postnatal period?
- Did the landlord know that the woman was pregnant?
  (Sometimes families were only allowed to rent on the grounds of 'no babies': couples would be evicted when the woman delivered.)
- Did the landlord agree to a confinement taking place in his premises?
- Were they in arrears with their rent? If so, were they likely to be evicted for non-payment before delivery?

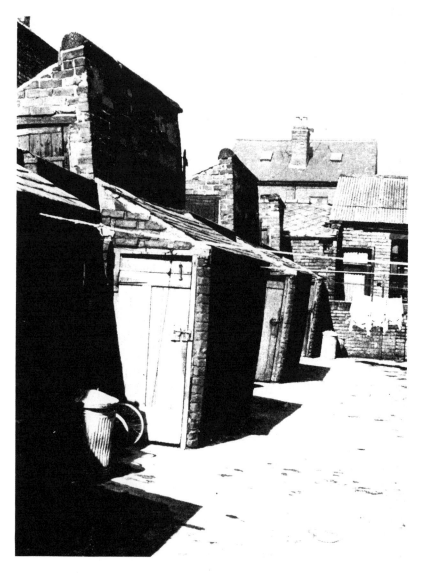

Figure 2.1 (including figures on pp. 49–50) most home births took place in the deprived inner-city areas of Nottingham.

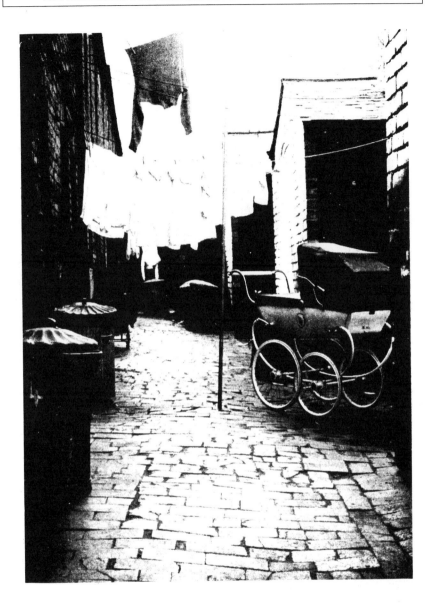

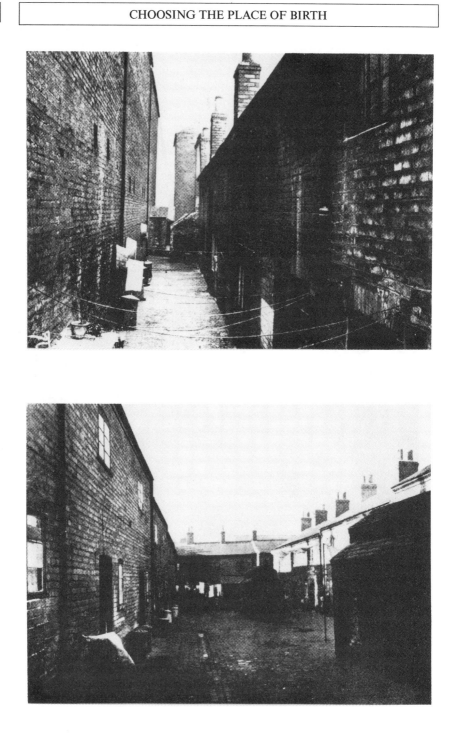

- Was the accommodation, bed and bedding 'reasonably' clean?
  (Such women never had a washing machine and seldom any means of boiling their washing, although in the inner-city areas there were 'wash houses' still in operation until the 1970s.)

The pressure for hospital beds on social grounds constantly exceeded the number available. There were 763 applications in 1962, of which 410 were granted (City of Nottingham 1962/26). The Medical Officer failed to acknowledge that 353 women who were not granted hospital beds were returned to their district midwife to be delivered at home, in a home which had already been identified as unsuitable. Thus of the 3323 home births in the city in 1962, 353 (11%) took place in home conditions which had been identified by the district midwife as unsuitable for home birth.

Nellie, a retired Supervisor of Midwives who had the thankless task of deciding to whom these beds should be allocated, shared these recollections:

> They used to have such things as 'social beds'. It was part of my job to go and vet them. The midwife used to vet them first, there wasn't any criteria really – for home delivery, what it amounted to was if the mother and father had a bedroom to themselves, even if they were sharing a terraced house with another family, they were put down for a home delivery. You couldn't make demands about inside toilets and running hot water, because more didn't have it than did.
>
> We used to put them down [for a social bed]. If the midwife said the home was not suitable we knew it was beyond the pale, these were usually the really dirty houses, and so we put them down for a social booking, but about half didn't get one.

Photographs shown on pages 48–50, taken during the period in question, illustrate some of the inner-city areas of Nottingham. During the years 1953–65, 10 538 recommendations were received by the local authority, of which 6795 were granted. The 3743 women who were refused a bed were returned to the care of the district midwife who had recommended a hospital booking on social grounds. Many women who were delivered at home during the period of the study had been identified as having unsuitable social or domestic circumstances; the responsibility lay with the district midwife to ensure that those shortcomings were resolved before labour commenced at home. This might entail the midwife in negotiations with the housing department to fumigate the house, the electricity board to reconnect a disconnected supply, or begging the local coal merchant to deliver coal when no payment could be expected. Layettes for babies were provided by the Women's Royal Voluntary Service, on the recommendation of the district midwife.

In their 1973 study for the National Children's Bureau, Wedge and Prosser examined the effect of social disadvantage on the children of

Britain. While indicating that there was no general agreement about what constituted social disadvantage, they argued that three factors were fundamentally important:

- family composition, i.e. large number of children in the family or one parent family;
- low income;
- poor housing.

(Wedge and Prosser 1973: 11)

The report showed that 'socially disadvantaged children suffered adversity in all aspects of life. This included their health, wealth, housing and education and as a result were smaller, sicker, less educated with less prospects in life than children of "ordinary families".'

They disclosed that one in ten of all 'disadvantaged' mothers made fewer than five antenatal attendances in pregnancy. One in 40 made no booking for delivery compared to one in 250 of 'ordinary' families (Wedge and Prosser 1973: 22). Over the years of this study, such women were well represented among those who delivered at home in Nottingham.

SELECTION PROCESS FOR PLACE OF BIRTH IN NOTTINGHAM

Women attended either their GP or district midwife for booking; the trend to first attendance with the GP increased over time. District midwives were instructed to urge women to attend a doctor (see Appendix A, Instructions to Midwives, paragraph 7). Selection for the place of birth could be made by either midwife or GP, although non-emergency referral would usually be made by the GP. Selection of the place of birth was governed by the availability of hospital beds, gestation at booking and social class.

BOOKING FOR A LOCAL AUTHORITY HOME BIRTH

Women came to be booked for home birth by several means:

- They chose a home birth with the district midwife and referred themselves directly to her home or the midwives' booking clinic.
- They had no particular preference for place of birth; the GP referred them to the district midwife for home booking.
- They attended the GP in early pregnancy with a view to a hospital birth, and were told they had no 'risk factor' for hospital birth and were referred to the district midwife for home booking.

- They had a risk factor but had attended the GP too late to secure a bed and were referred to the district midwife for home booking.
- They had been referred to the hospital on medical/obstetric grounds by the district midwife or GP and sent back to the midwife for home booking, due to insufficient hospital beds.
- They had applied for a social emergency bed through the local authority and been rejected and returned to the district midwife for home booking (see Application for hospital bed on social grounds page 46).
- Oral evidence indicates that some of the 'socially disadvantaged' women and grande multiparae who wanted home birth did not book until late pregnancy to avoid hospital booking.

In effect, district midwives booked women who chose a home birth and all those who could not be fitted into the system elsewhere. In recalling the difficulty of getting beds for women who desperately needed them Olga described an incident in 1962:

> I remember taking a white unmarried girl to see the consultant for booking and being turned away: no beds. This girl was very anaemic, unsupported, tiny room on Dame Agnes Street, no heating. Anyway I remember saying to her not to worry, when she went into labour, I would say the fetal heart was unstable and admit her as an emergency. I did that more than once.

Home booking was confirmed by the GP who signed the 'fitness for inhalation analgesia' form and a home assessment visit from the midwife. This was in one sense academic, as so many of the women had already been turned down for a social emergency bed. As another midwife said:

> It was a complete farce, no-one in my patch had a proper bathroom or inside lav ... a lot of them in the back to backs were still sharing a single outside cold water tap and lav ... between 6 houses ... and I did more than 600 home deliveries down there [that part of the city].

BOOKING FOR A HOSPITAL BIRTH

There is no question that women with severe medical complications, such as heart disease and diabetes, were referred for hospital booking, except for those who refused to go or whose pregnancy went undiagnosed. Women who developed severe obstetric problems in pregnancy would also be referred for consultant opinion. However, the extent of the problem of bed shortage or of their allocation to women who had no indications for hospital birth cannot be overstated. There are examples in the midwives' registers of hospital or home-booked women who, following diagnosis of intrauterine fetal death (IUFD), had been sent home from hospital to wait up to a week (due to bed shortage) for a hospital bed for induction of labour to deliver the dead fetus. On occasions they went into labour at home and sent for the district midwife who delivered the macerated fetus at home. Any such stillbirths were attributed to home birth statistics.

A retired midwife had this to say:

> It made me very angry ... I sent one of my patients to hospital because she was small for dates ... it took them 3 weeks to see her ... then they sent her back with a note ... she'd got an IUFD ... they couldn't admit her for induction for five days ... she was heartbroken ... I went round that night and did a membrane sweep ... by midnight it was all over ... she'd delivered at home.

There are also examples where an obstetrician, because of bed shortage, came on to the district and performed procedures at home (see page 98, multiple births). Again, any deaths contributed to the home still-birth rate. It was a regular occurrence for an obstetrician to undertake inductions at home to avoid admission, for severe postmaturity, of home-booked women into the maternity hospital which was already bursting at the seams.

Women who had no 'risk' factors were not excluded from hospital booking: the secret was to attend the GP as early as possible in pregnancy and get referred to the hospital before the quota for the month in which they were due was filled. The maternity-bed shortage was so well known to the public that the local joke ran: 'to get a bed in hospital you have to book three months before you get pregnant'.

Apparently, many women who gave birth in hospital could by their criteria and home circumstances have been delivered at home; 67% of hospital-booked women who sustained a BBA at home fell outside of criteria for a home birth; or, put another way, 33% were apparently suitable for home birth (see page 95). It is not possible to say from available data what percentage of women booked for hospital birth were suitable for home birth by the 1967 criteria. However, if the BBA example of 33% of women booked for hospital birth being suitable for home birth were true across all the births in the study, then it is possible that thousands of women who fell outside the criteria for home birth but were not delivered at home, could have been delivered in hospital if 'safety' had been the major objective of hospital delivery.

Newson and Newson found in their 1960 survey in the City of Nottingham that overall, 26% of primigravidae were delivered at home; but while 18% of social class one and two first-time mothers had a home birth, 31% of social class three and 22% of social class four gave birth to their first baby at home. Similarly, the same study showed that for later births, while 59% of social class one and two mothers gave birth at home, 83% of social class five babies were home deliveries (Newson and Newson 1963: 165–7).

They also found that unofficial discrimination was being exercised by GPs to send more middle-class mothers to the single-purpose NHS maternity hospital, which was described by the mothers as 'posh'. 49% of social class one and two first-time mothers were delivered in the maternity hospital and 14% of social class five while 71% of social class five were delivered in the wards of the general or women's hospital and 31% of social class one and two. For later births, 6% of social class one returned to the maternity hospital but none of social class five women were delivered of later babies in the maternity hospital.

It was identified that nationally the link between criteria and the process of selection for place of birth was tenuous; home bookings were markedly weighted towards women described as being in the 'lower social classes', despite evidence of the risk of higher perinatal mortality in this group (Butler and Bonham 1963: 289). This finding was reflected in the place of birth for residents of the City of Nottingham (Goodacre 1974: 139; Newson and Newson 1963: 24–5 and 164–8). An assumption could be made that this would unfavourably affect outcomes to mother and baby for home birth; however, the findings of Chapter 4, do not support that assumption. While some authorities with adequate hospital and domiciliary mid-wifery facilities could encourage women to make choices freely, Nottingham should, on the face of it, have been unable to offer this service to women from any social class.

CONTINUITY AND CHOICE FOR WOMEN IN NOTTINGHAM

Women who chose a home birth were fortunate in that there was an efficient and safe domiciliary midwifery service, with a local midwife prepared to book and care for them. Midwives' district registers and booking sheets indicate that as many as 90% of women who were eventually delivered at home presented themselves for home booking as their first choice. In the last analysis, all who chose a home birth and all who could not be accommodated elsewhere were delivered at home.

However, there were women who wished for or needed a maternity bed and were unable to secure one; and those, often the grande multiparae, who were referred to an obstetrician against their wishes. Despite the biased selection process and the disregard of the criteria for the place of birth, it appears from Goodacre's study at the end of the period that women in Nottingham generally gave birth to their babies in the place they chose (Goodacre 1974: 139).

In contrast, the Office of Population, Census and Survey's survey, *Women's Experience of Maternity Care*, undertaken in Nottingham in 1991, indicated that while 99% of Nottingham's babies were born in a consultant unit, 50% of the 1074 women who were surveyed after delivery said they wished they had been given information about domino births and 27% had wished for information about home births (Allison 1991: 53).

END OF AN ERA: INTEGRATING AND CENTRALIZING MIDWIFERY SERVICES

A recommendation of the Report of the Maternity Services Committee (Cranbrook Report) (HMSO 1959) was for an integrated midwifery service: that is, a single midwifery service across the hospital and local authority management barrier. This was not possible in employment terms until the 1968 Health Services and Public Health Act (HMSO 1968), which gave licence to domiciliary midwives to practise in hospital as well as 'on the district'.

Nevertheless, during the years between Cranbrook and Peel (HMSO 1970), the future provision of midwifery services was subject of much political and professional debate. It was also the cause of friction between hospital and domiciliary midwives. As the argument against home birth grew in strength, in reverse proportions the image and authority of district midwives diminished. Their role had become associated with non-interventionist 'normal' practice, when the conventional wisdom was for hospitalization and intervention in childbirth to improve maternal and infant mortality outcomes.

Hospital-based midwifery services were overstretched and pressure grew greater as more births were directed for hospital delivery. Managers expected that the 'over-staffing' of domiciliary midwifery services as the home-birth rate plummeted would be redirected to alleviate pressure on the new maternity units. In reality there was no 'over-staffing' in the community. As the home-birth rate dropped in Nottingham, the number of domiciliary midwives was reduced by natural wastage and other posts reduced to part-time, despite the historic under-resourcing. As hospital births grew in number, so did the number of early discharges, thus maintaining district midwives' workloads. By 1976 a 'domino' midwifery service had been introduced, which further called upon community resources. Nationally, the debate threatened to divide the profession between hospital and district-based midwives. In 1967 the *Midwives Chronicle and Nursing Notes*, offered a forum for the discussion. The two points of view were hotly debated over a number of weeks and could best be summarized in the following correspondence:

The hospital-employed midwives' opinion

It would seem to be of benefit to everyone concerned if all midwives were brought together under one administrative body. The coverage of duties could be arranged as four shifts morning, afternoon, night duty, domiciliary work. All deliveries to be conducted in hospital and discharged if satisfactory at 48 hours. Domiciliary coverage from hospital ... to cover any mother requiring home confinement.

All staff would be able to take part in clinic work, labour-room work, ante- and postnatal care and domiciliary care.

Advantages to the patient:

- full antenatal care in home and clinic and not get so much differing advice;
- delivered in hospital with full coverage for emergencies;
- would probably know the midwife who delivered her;
- could still be delivered at home if she so wished;
- only one centre to phone for a midwife;
- the midwife would be up-to-date in her professional knowledge and skills.

Advantages to the midwife:

- no midwife would have to be on call, as at present, in local authority service;
- all midwives would be able to practise midwifery in all its aspects;
- all midwives would be able to retain their individuality;
- all midwives would benefit from practising in units where modern methods and techniques are practised.

It is obvious that any proposals will be met with varying opinions, but the patient and her needs must be of prime importance to us all.

The domiciliary midwives' view

In modern times we all like to choose what to wear, where to spend our holidays, so – why not – most important of all – where to have our babies?

Domiciliary midwives today are very much up-to-date with modern facilities, sterile packs, disposable gloves, and syringes, flying squad, patient's records for HBs and investigation for the Rh factor, parentcraft, relaxation and the relief of pain.

Homes today are also up-to-date. With government grants, nearly all have hot and cold water, heated bathrooms as well as bedrooms, telephones, etc.

With all mod. cons. a mother should be allowed to stay at home if she chooses, and not bullied or frightened into going into hospital. Quite often after a [hospital] antenatal visit a mother is distressed and very confused, because she is told she is safer in hospital. Her anxieties build up to a mountain of fear, and at the onset of labour she is totally unprepared mentally. As trained midwives we all know only too well the serious consequences.

Surely without doubt, if we are to give our mothers and babies the service they deserve, there must be a domiciliary service.

(Midwives Chronicle and Nursing Notes,
December 1967/416)

In most ways these two letters, written almost 30 years ago, summarize both the dilemma within the profession and contemporary conventional wisdom about 'place of birth' and women's right to choose. So great was the dissension within the profession that district midwives sought peer support within the domiciliary midwives forum of the Royal College of Midwives, as to a great extent they felt both marginalized and threatened. Indeed, the letter from the hospital midwife clearly implies that the knowledge and practices of domiciliary midwives were out-of-date, and by implication 'unsafe'. And certainly this seems to imply an analogy between hospital birth and safety.

At the British Medical Association's annual meeting in July 1963, obstetricians recommended that the government should launch: 'a crash programme of new maternity hospital units, otherwise mothers and their children might be in peril ... a grave emergency' (Mason 1963: 10).

By 1973, Nottingham had opened the first of its centralized maternity units. Although it was not possible to open all the wards for some time due to lack of midwifery staff, those from the soon-to-close small units were reluctant to transfer and by 1972 the newly appointed management team had to employ 24 'agency midwives' in order to open the new facility.

In a survey, all 192 women in Nottingham who had home births in 1980 and 1981 and a similar group who had hospital births were questioned about their experience and future plans for birth. One finding was that 12% of women delivered in hospital expressed the view that they would have a home birth next time. The authors concluded that if this was considered in absolute terms as a percentage of the 19 177 births in the City in the two-year period, then this indicated that 2300 of the women who gave birth in hospital would prefer home birth next time (Caplan and Madeley 1985: 307–13). By this time there was no longer a universally available home birth service.

CHOOSING THE PLACE OF BIRTH

Key points

- Nottingham lagged behind the rest of the country in moving towards hospitalization of birth, due to shortage of maternity beds. Consequently home-birth data is available for a longer time frame than the rest of the country; that data is central to this project.
- Choices of place of birth and carer in Nottingham were: NHS maternity beds in general hospitals and one single-purpose maternity hospital, local authority home births, private maternity hospitals, doctors and independent midwives. Over time, the demand for private doctors and midwives disappeared.
- Until 1964, more than 50% of births in Nottingham occurred at home.
- In 1967, the Ministry of Health issued criteria for normal (home) confinement. It is likely that some 52% of women, throughout the period of the study, who delivered at home in Nottingham did not fulfil these criteria; this calls into question the long-held assumption that women who were delivered at home were low risk for complication.
- An annual quota of hospital beds was made for women with poor domestic or social conditions. During the period 1953 to 1965, 3745 such women, deemed to be at risk, were refused a hospital bed and delivered at home.
- There is evidence that there was a bias towards home birth for women described as being in the 'lower social classes', and a bias towards birth in the one maternity hospital for women of social classes one and two.

Transfers in and out of domiciliary care

3

In the last chapter we considered the place of birth, including how and why women came to be delivered at home. In this chapter we come to quite the most complex issue regarding the place of birth debate: that of the transfer of women in and out of domiciliary care. In effect, this chapter could be seen as a rather complicated jigsaw puzzle. There is no means of recreating with absolute accuracy an exact account of the transfers between home and hospital. However, using all the data available from the Medical Officer of Health Reports it is possible to show the number of antenatal transfers from home to hospital. Furthermore with the additional data from the midwives' registers and some deduction and calculation, it is possible to estimate the likely extent of transfers between place of birth in labour. All available information has been used in putting together this elaborated account of transfers in and out of domiciliary care.

For the past 30 years there has been a belief that, during this period, the transfer of care between home and hospital was a one-way phenomenon which caused hospital outcomes alone to be unfavourably skewed by the high mortality of cases originally booked for home but later transferred to hospital care (Butler and Bonham 1963: 288). City of Nottingham data reveals that this is not as straightforward as was assumed. When we explore the issue of how many home-booked women in Nottingham were transferred to hospital care antenatally and in labour, and the way in which hospital-booked and unbooked women were delivered at home and counted in home birth statistics, a different picture emerges.

Thus the question asked here is: how many women who were booked for home birth went on to be delivered at home and how many women who were delivered at home were booked for home birth? We further explore how women came to be delivered in a place other than their booked place of birth and what effect this movement of women between place of birth might have had on perinatal and maternal mortality statistics.

Apart from those who did not present themselves for antenatal care, most women chose or were streamlined into hospital or home booking soon after they presented for antenatal care (see preceding chapter). Once allocated into a system of care, that remained as their intended place of birth unless they were formally transferred out again.

However, some women were transferred between systems of care, and some were never booked for care and had to be fitted into the system when labour commenced or birth took place. Thus transfers in and out of domiciliary care occurred both during the antenatal period and around the time of birth. Using data published in the Annual Reports of the Medical Officer of Health, the following table of antenatal transfers from home to hospital of city residents during 1948–68 has been devised.

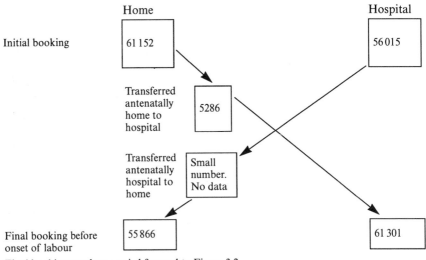

Final booking numbers carried forward to Figure 3.2

Figure 3.1 Antenatal transfers of place of booking – City of Nottingham residents 1948–68

For the purpose of this exercise, the antenatal period is defined as the time from first booking up until, but not including, the onset of labour. Of women booked for home delivery, 5286 (8.6%) were transferred to hospital booking in this period. The purpose of transfer was believed to be to improve the possibility of a good outcome to mother and/or baby following the diagnosis of a complication. This data was published routinely until 1968, although detail of the reasons for transfer was not monitored.

Women were transferred from home to hospital booking for medical, obstetric and social reasons. As previously discussed on page 45, many women who did not fulfil the criteria for a home confinement were booked at home because of the shortage of hospital beds. Medical and obstetric reasons for transfer included gestational diabetes, antepartum haemorrhage, severe hypertension, multiple pregnancy, premature labour and suspected fetal abnormality.

Some women whose social/domestic conditions were unsatisfactory were referred directly for a hospital bed on social grounds, usually by the midwife, and were not transfers from home to hospital in the antenatal period. Some were booked for home delivery and only when the midwife made her home-assessment visit did it become apparent that the home was not suitable. In such cases, the woman would be referred for a social emergency bed and if her application was successful her booking would be a transfer from home to hospital delivery in the antenatal period. Other women who booked for home delivery experienced changed circumstances in pregnancy. For example, she may have separated from her husband and no longer have suitable accommodation or support, or the family may have been evicted for non-payment of rent. There were, of course, many other circumstances which could give rise to the need for a social booking, after booking for home birth. Such cases were referred for antenatal transfer to hospital booking on social grounds and not all of them would be successful. Of the 61 152 women booked for home birth between 1948 and 1968, 5286 (8.6%) were transferred for hospital booking.

The registers show that a few women changed their booking from hospital to home in the antenatal period, sometimes following marriage to the father of the baby, or when they had been allocated a council house. Sometimes they simply changed their mind about where they wanted the baby to be born. Occasionally they had medical conditions which warranted hospital birth and continuously defaulted on their hospital appointments until the district midwife decided that it was better to have a planned home confinement to which she would be invited, than a planned hospital booking which the woman had no intention of keeping. The number of times that reasons are given in the registers for transfer from hospital to home booking are few. The numbers of such transfers are small and add nothing to the sum of this debate, other than recognition of the fact that they sometimes occurred.

LIKELY EXTENT OF CHANGE OF PLACE OF BIRTH

The extent to which women were transferred between the place of birth in labour, especially those who were hospital booked or unbooked and delivered at home, was not intentionally monitored. However, using what data there is and evidence from the midwives' registers, with a certain amount of detective work, analysis and ingenuity it is possible to give an estimated exposition of the extent and circumstance of the change of place of birth in labour. The following table seeks to explain that the movement of women in labour was not simply a one-way process between home and hospital. The information is for the period 1948–68. After 1968, relevant data was no longer published in the Medical Officer of Health Reports.

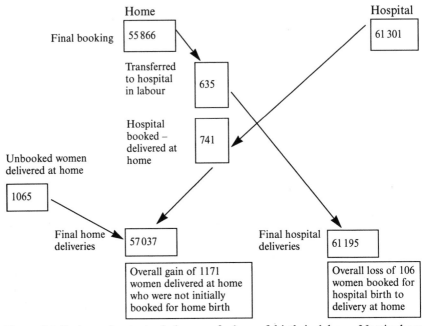

Figure 3.2 Estimated extent of change of place of birth in labour, Nottingham 1948–68

On page 70 the chart shown above is elaborated, drawing upon the statistical and estimated data evidence that follows. The data demonstrate that far from there being a gain to the hospital statistics of women booked for home birth but transferred to hospital, there was most likely an overall loss of women booked for hospital to delivery at home. There was also a further large gain to the home confinement statistics of women who were unbooked and had had no antenatal care and who delivered at home. A number of these women were transferred to hospital following delivery, but the birth was counted in home statistics as was any subsequent outcome to mother or baby. A few of these women were transferred to hospital in labour, often via the emergency obstetric service (for discussion see page 66–7).

In order to draw conclusions from Nottingham data about transfers in and out of domiciliary care it is necessary to understand how many and by what means women were transferred between the place of birth at or around the time of labour. The results are summarized in Table 3.2 on page 70.

MEANS BY WHICH WOMEN WERE TRANSFERRED BETWEEN PLACE OF BIRTH AT LABOUR

There were a number of means by which women were transferred or came to be delivered in a place other than where they had booked at labour. These were:

- obstetric emergency team (flying squad);
- midwife admissions in labour (from home to hospital, of home, hospital or unbooked women);
- delivery of unbooked women at home;
- unintended delivery of hospital booked women at home.

OBSTETRIC EMERGENCY TEAM (FLYING SQUAD)

In the years 1949 to 1967 the MOH kept data on the obstetric emergency team. There were 51 985 home births; the flying squad attended 545 district emergencies. While many of the women were booked for home birth, some were booked for hospital or unbooked. Obstetric emergencies were 1.0% of total home births; put another way, the flying squad attended on average one call every two weeks, or each midwife called the squad approximately once a year.

Attendance by the obstetric emergency team did not mean that women were admitted to hospital; in the majority of cases of home-booked women, in the early years of the study, the mother or baby were treated at home and left to the care of the district midwife and GP, with no recorded ill effects. As one of the midwives who worked during the late 1940s recalled:

It seemed that the poorer they were ... the more babies they had the less likely they were to agree to a hospital confinement ... if they bled after delivery (postpartum haemorrhage) ... or got a retained placenta it was all the worse because so many of them were verging on malnutrition because of the war ... giving all their rations to the little ones ... a lot of them had bad anaemia in those days ... but the flying squad came out and gave them a transfusion and they stayed at home ... none the worse for it ... we looked after them well.

Another district midwife recalled:

> My only experience of calling the flying squad was to my first home delivery as a qualified midwife. I was called to the house of a woman who was unbooked ... no antenatal care although she was rhesus negative ... second pregnancy. She had delivered four hours before ... in a cold house, no running water ... retained placenta ... blood loss about 2000 ml. The baby weighed 10lb 12ozs and still lay between the mother's thighs ... cold and shocked ... like the mother. On examination, she had a third degree tear. I called the flying squad, delivered the placenta, controlled the bleeding, made sure the baby was breathing and wrapped it in my warm coat as there was no heating in the house ... they were both OK in the end.

In many ways the circumstances of these incidents demonstrate the range of social and economic factors which were instrumental in hampering the overall improvement in maternal and perinatal mortality statistics in the period in question.

Table 3.1 Reasons for the 545 calls to the obstetric flying squad in Nottingham

Reason for call	Number
Primary and secondary PPH	170
Retained placenta/shock	280
Antepartum haemorrhage	22
Malpresentation 2nd twin	8
Eclampsia (unbooked women)	5
Abortion	3
Prolapsed cord	3
Asphyxia baby	4
Uterine inertia	1
Anaemia	1
Fetal distress	11
Delay 2nd stage	1
Ruptured uterus	1
Unknown causes	35
Total calls	545

Source: City of Nottingham Medical Officer of Health Reports 1949–67

There is no way of determining which of the above were booked for home, hospital or unbooked (except in the case of women with eclampsia where a record was kept indicating that all were unbooked), and which were transferred to hospital and which kept at home. However, the overwhelming majority of calls were to women who were already delivered; or in cases such as malpresentation and prolapsed cord would most likely have been delivered at home after the arrival of the obstetric team. Thus the birth, whatever the place of booking or outcome, would have been attributed to domiciliary statistics.

In the 19-year period there were 11 cases of fetal distress, three of prolapsed cord and four of asphyxia of the baby, for which the emergency team was called, and it is evident from the midwives' registers that a proportion were hospital booked or unbooked.

It is probable that the number of times the obstetric emergency team was called to assist at a home-booked birth resulting in transfer in labour of a case with a negative outcome for the infant, reflected in hospital birth statistics; this was offset by the number of occasions on which a hospital booked or unbooked case was delivered at home with a negative effect to home-birth statistics.

Given that it is not possible to establish the intended place of birth, except for all the cases of eclampsia, which were unbooked, and that so few of these cases would have affected infant mortality in terms of skewing either hospital or home statistics, no account of them has been taken in this analysis. Indeed, it is not possible to establish whether the five women with eclampsia were delivered before or after arrival at hospital.

MIDWIFE ADMISSIONS IN LABOUR

Under an arrangement with the obstetricians, city midwives were able to make direct admissions of women who developed a complication in labour. During the years 1952 to 1968, the medical officer of health recorded these admissions. No details of cause, circumstance or outcome was kept however. City midwives admitted 526 women in labour (see Table 3.2 page 70), an average of one admission per midwife per year, or 1.1% of home births in the period. It is likely that some of these women were home booked. However, it is apparent from the midwives' registers that some were hospital booked or unbooked (see unbooked cases attended by city midwives, below, and stillbirths page 91). However, for the purposes of this debate an assumption has been made that all such transfers were of home-booked women and the statistics both real and estimated in the 'elaborated' chart on page 70 are based on that premise.

DELIVERY OF UNBOOKED WOMEN AT HOME

Unbooked women who requested maternity assistance at or around the time of labour were attended by the district midwife or very occasionally by the general practitioner. Admissions to hospital were only made via the domiciliary service, and only if there was an obstetric or social reason. Thus unbooked cases were almost exclusively the responsibility of the district midwife, and would only be transferred to hospital at her request. Any such transfers are included in either 'Obstetric emergency team transfers' (page 65–6) or 'Midwife admissions in labour' (page 67). The overwhelming majority were BBAs delivered at home and counted in home-birth statistics. Indeed the District Midwife issued the birth notification to her Authority and Local Registrar of births.

From 1949 to 1956 the Medical Officer of Health kept a record of unbooked home deliveries attended at or around the time of delivery by district midwives: the total for the eight-year period was 367. Of the 20 837 home births in this period, the percentage of unbooked cases remained constant at around 1.8% per annum of total home births (see page 70). Unbooked cases delivered at home were registered and counted in the statistics for home birth; Campbell, Macdonald, Macfarlane *et al.* in their 1979 study published in 1984 demonstrated a near 50-fold variation in perinatal mortality outcomes between those booked for home delivery and those who were unbooked. (see page 96.) Most would have resulted in birth before the arrival of the district midwife (BBA, see page 93). In other cases the woman or relative would have called the midwife when labour was established and it is very likely that such women would have been delivered at home.

Murphy, Daumey, Gray *et al.* (1984: 1429), Tew (1995) and Campbell et al. (1984) have illustrated the rise over time in the proportion of unplanned to planned births occurring at home. The registers of the midwives and the oral evidence of the Supervisor of Midwives reinforce this view. Therefore the estimated figure in the elaborated chart on page 70 is a conservative estimate composed of the 367 (1.8%) of cases known to have occurred between 1949 and 1956 and 1.8% of total births for the period during which the Medical Officer did not publish these statistics.

Women who were unbooked, with no antenatal care, had BBAs for a number of reasons: they often wanted a home birth and knew that their medical or social contraindications were such that they would be referred to hospital. Sometimes they simply wanted to avoid the censure they felt they would receive from the medical authority for being pregnant. Although the following example did not culminate in a BBA, it is a perfect illustration of the circumstances which decided women to resist booking:

Mrs James, a lively young woman of 23, had a slipped disc; her first baby had been born prematurely and died after a few hours. She had been told she mustn't have any more children, 'They said I couldn't stand the weight of carrying. Well, I was determined to have a baby, so I said to Jack, "We'll just go ahead and have one and we won't tell anyone or ask anyone's advice." So we did. I never saw any doctor or clinic or anyone right through until I called the midwife … he was 10lbs … I wouldn't have missed it for the world'.

(Newson and Newson 1963: 19)

This clearly illustrates that the responsibility for unbooked cases fell to the district midwife, and even though she was not called until the onset of labour, birth took place at home. Other women who regularly resisted booking were the grande multips, who felt that every booking for delivery would be accompanied by medical disapproval and advice that they should be sterilized in the immediate post-partum period. Those who accepted hospital booking to have surgical sterilization within the first week frequently absconded from the hospital within 48 hours. Most simply avoided conflict with authority by not having care, except to send for the district midwife during labour or after the birth.

Some women, who were obese or menopausal, did not know they were pregnant until the birth took place. Other BBAs occurred to young frightened girls who concealed their pregnancies, and a few to women who were described in the registers as 'educationally subnormal'. The estimated figures for unbooked women delivered at home is elaborated on page 70.

UNINTENDED DELIVERY OF HOSPITAL-BOOKED WOMEN AT HOME

From registers and oral evidence it is clear that hospital-booked women delivered at home often through precipitate labour. Sometimes they were visiting from another area and a district midwife would attend when a relative called for help.

Some who were booked for hospital deliberately called no one in labour as they had been booked into hospital against their wishes, due to medical or social reasons. They ensured a home birth by having an unattended birth and then calling for the midwife, who would often keep them at home after the birth.

From the registers of the district midwives, using the total sample of 11 850 (19%) of total births in the city in the period, 1.3% of women delivered at home were booked for hospital delivery. The sample includes deliveries from across the time range and of midwives who worked across the geographical spread of the city. Thus in the absence of any other evidence, the number of deliveries assumed to have been booked for hospital but delivered at home is calculated on the basis of 1.3% of all deliveries over the whole period (see page 70).

ELABORATION AND CONCLUSION OF TRANSFERS IN AND OUT OF DOMICILIARY CARE

The issue of antenatal transfer is clear: 5286 women (8.6% of women booked for home birth in the period) were transferred from home to hospital booking in the antenatal period and a small, unknown number were transferred from hospital to home. The purpose of transfer was to improve the possibility of a good outcome to mother and/or baby following the diagnosis of a medical, obstetric or social complication. There is no means of checking the outcome of these transfers, other than those which appear in the registers of the midwives included in this study.

THE EXTENT OF TRANSFERS BETWEEN HOME AND HOSPITAL AND THE LIKELY EXTENT OF DELIVERY OF UNBOOKED AND HOSPITAL-BOOKED WOMEN AT HOME

The evidence from the Annual Health Committee Reports of the Medical Officer of Health from 1948 to 1968 and the data from the registers of the district midwives puts a different slant on the notion that hospital statistics alone were skewed by births not planned to occur there. The table below has been compiled to elaborate the summary Figure 3.2 on page 64 showing the likely extent of the shift of women between the place of birth at or around the time of labour, drawing upon the evidence presented in this chapter.

Table 3.2   Likely extent of change of place of birth in labour Nottingham 1948–68 (elaboration of chart on page 64)

Final hospital bookings	**61 301**
Final home bookings	**55 866**
Midwife admissions in labour Actual 1952–68 = 526 (see p. 67) estimated at 1.1% of total births for 1948–51 = 109	**635**
Unbooked delivered at home Actual 1949–56 = 367 (see p. 67) Unbkd del. at home, estimated at 1.8% of total births for 1948 and 1957–68 = 698	**1065**
Hosp bkd del. at home calculated as 1.3% of total home births 1948–68 (see p. 69)	**741**
Total delivered in hospital (actual)	**61 195**
Total delivered at home (actual)	**57 037**

Source: City of Nottingham Medical Officer of Health Reports 1948–68 and personal registers of district midwives.

It is likely that 635 women were transferred from home to hospital in labour by city midwives. Many were booked for home birth, but some were booked for hospital or unbooked for care in any place. It is these women who, it has been argued, have skewed the statistics for maternal and infant mortality outcomes in hospital. On the other hand it is likely that some 1806 women, 741 of whom were hospital booked and 1065 who were unbooked, with their enormously higher risk of perinatal mortality, were delivered at home.

Goodacre (1974: 140) writing retrospectively of perinatal outcomes in Nottingham said:

> The hospital rate (perinatal death) was nearly four times as great as the domiciliary rate but this is probably explained by the fact that a greater proportion of difficult cases are confined in hospital. Indeed, it could be argued that the rate for domiciliary confinements, although considerably lower than for hospitals, is nevertheless too high, since only relatively normal cases should be confined at home.

The evidence in this chapter does not support Goodacre's statement nor the belief that the transfer of care between home and hospital was a one-way phenomenon causing hospital mortality outcomes alone to be unfavourably skewed by the high mortality rate of cases originally booked for home and later transferred to hospital. If the analysis of this data is read in conjunction with the knowledge that it is similarly likely that more than 50% of women delivered at home in Nottingham did not fulfil the criteria for home birth, it becomes difficult to maintain the arguments which ultimately shifted government policy towards 100% hospital birth.

TRANSFERS IN AND OUT OF DOMICILIARY CARE

Key points

- Between 1948 and 1968 in Nottingham, 5286 (8.6% of women booked for home birth in the period) were transferred to hospital booking in the antenatal period for medical, obstetric and social reasons.
- Of the 51 985 births occurring at home between 1949 and 1967 the emergency obstetric team attended on 545 occasions. Some cases were hospital booked or unbooked.
- The majority of women for whom the emergency obstetric team was called were already delivered; thus the birth and its outcome would be attributed to home-birth statistics.
- In the period 1952–68 city midwives admitted 526 (1.1%) women directly to hospital; this was equivalent to one admission per midwife per year. Some of these women were hospital booked or unbooked.
- This study lends weight to previous evidence which refutes the long-held belief that hospital statistics alone were skewed by high-risk births which were not planned to occur there. In the period 1948–68 an estimated 1806 women who had had no antenatal care and were unbooked for a place of birth, or were hospital booked, were delivered at home, compared to 635 women who were home, hospital or unbooked and transferred to hospital from home in labour.

Home confinement: outcomes and experiences

4

How could you help pregnant women if you didn't know them ... if you didn't go to their house and meet the old man [husband] and see what they were up against ... when you'd done that ... you knew how to help them ... it might have been ... simple ... sending for the plumber ... but if you'd got no money and no telephone ... that was easier said than done.

(Audrey)

The mothers, babies and families of Nottingham are as much a part of this study as the midwives who cared for them. From this distance in time it is not easy to judge how these families viewed the care they received or the options that were offered. In many ways there is no true comparison with today's family or society. Families were larger in the early part of the study and there was little unemployment for those in Nottingham who wished to and were capable of work. But in real terms the working-class family income did not support home ownership, family cars and foreign holidays as it does today.

The expectation of the average maternity service user in terms of consultation, decision-making, choice or control in place of birth and carer was much less than would be the case today. Family planning was not generally freely available and among some of the women in this study pregnancy, birth and abortion, both accidental and criminal, were a monotonous and wearying aspect of life in which they had no aesthetic interest. Today, birth is more commonly a planned experience which happens only occasionally in most families and women and their partners demand a great deal of control in terms of choice of place of birth, type of birth and carer.

In this chapter we look at the mothers of Nottingham and the babies who were delivered at home. We examine something of the process of home confinement and the statistical outcomes. From previous chapters we understand how district midwives worked, that they practised as individuals within partnerships and that their workload was excessive. They offered continuity of carer and earned a high status in the community. In this chapter we explore the outcome of their work.

In statistical and descriptive terms the following issues, related to midwifery care in the City of Nottingham at some time between 1948 and 1972, are discussed: maternal death and stillbirth at home and hospital. The use of oxygen by district midwives and the incidence of multiple birth at home are examined, as is the care of low birthweight babies and breast-feeding rates among home births.

Charts, tables and statistical analyses in this chapter cover various periods of time, and different sets of the registers of the 14 midwives are used in some of the analyses. Explanations of these variations are given in each case. Where a time span less than 1948–72 is used it is entirely because the information was only available for the years indicated. In no instance has data published in the Medical Officer of Health Reports related to the immediate topic been omitted.

Similarly, all of the registers of the midwives have been used where they contained relevant information. However, not all the midwives worked throughout the whole period. On occasions where data from the Medical Officer of Health Reports is for a period less than the whole time, information from midwives' registers is used for the matching years. In some cases, information from the registers has been withheld, such as the exact year of some births, e.g. excerpts from the personal register, in order to avoid identifying the midwife or the mothers.

In terms of client satisfaction and women's experience of birth, there is much less evidence to draw upon. However, an attempt is made in this chapter to give context and texture to the women and babies whose birth experience comprise the data of this study. The illustration on page 75 shows some of Nottingham's mothers and toddlers outside Edwards Lane Welfare Clinic *c*. 1949. A midwives' clinic was held here once a week. The illustration on page 76 is a photograph taken by Joyce (district midwife), probably in the 1960s, of one of the inner-city streets that formed part of her patch, which was largely composed of similar streets.

During 1989, in the course of completing a Masters dissertation, I asked five women who had hospital births followed by home births in the 1960s how they compared those experiences. All said they preferred the home birth and stated that if they were to have another child they would still choose a home birth. Interestingly, each of these women had daughters who had given birth to children during the preceding few years, only one of whom had had a home birth. When questioned about this the women felt pleased that their daughters had given birth in hospital because they believed it was safer.

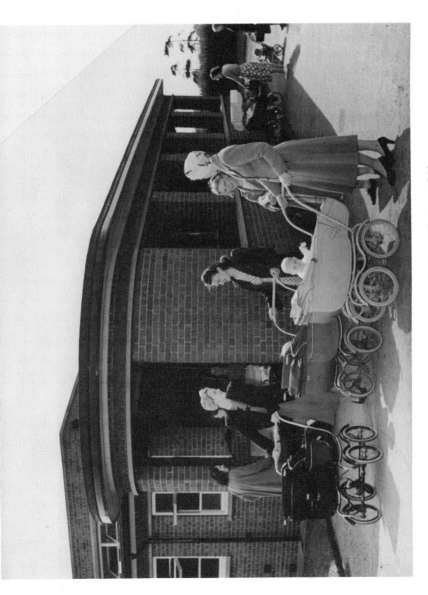

Figure 4.1 Mothers and babies outside Edwards Lane Welfare Clinic, c. 1949

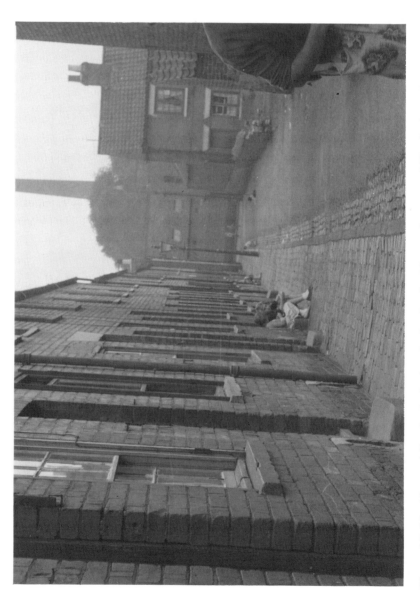

Figure 4.2 Most home deliveries took place in the deprived inner-city areas of Nottingham. (Reproduced with kind permission from Joyce Tarlton)

It is clear that these middle-aged mothers had come to believe the 'official discourse' that all birth was safest in hospital. Where they were being asked to consider the 'safety' of their daughter and grandchild they were swayed by protectiveness to put them in a 'safe' environment. However, when they were asked to consider an acceptable birth environment for themselves, it was clear that their priorities veered more towards comfort and aestheticism (Allison 1989: 35).

HOME CONFINEMENT

Until recently, birth at home was part of the culture of British society. Every childbearing woman knew something about home birth, whether or not it was an option they would choose. Mothers, grandmothers, neighbours or friends knew where the district midwife lived and the day and time of her clinic. Similarly, they knew what home confinement entailed. The district midwife booked women for home delivery and gave them the *Preparations for Home Confinement* list. Just one sheet of paper (see illustration page 78) told them all they needed to know about preparing for home delivery.

In their 1963 survey of 709 City of Nottingham mothers who were delivered at home and hospital, Newson and Newson had this to say about women's comments on their preference for home birth:

> For the mother at home there is none of this [impersonality of hospital]; she has the comforting familiarity of her own bed, or her own fireside until she reaches the second stage; some familiar person – her husband, her mother or a neighbour – will probably be there with her to rub her back; **and, above all, there will be the midwife, who will have examined her ... during her pregnancy**, and with whom, therefore, she already has a personal relationship. The midwife may be rushed off her feet; she may, in fact, have to dash back and forth between confinements; but she always seems able to provide that touch of intimacy, of real friendliness, which is of the greatest support to a woman in labour.
> *(Newson and Newson 1963: 25–6) (Author's emphasis)*

It is interesting that Newson and Newson picked up the themes that remain significant to women today. Continuity of carer, the importance of the role of the midwife and the need that some women have for the security of their own home in labour, seemed to be as relevant in the 1960s as they are today.

Part of the preparation was that the patient identified someone reliable to be with her in labour to help the midwife and to be available to help in the home in the 'lying-in period'. It was not necessarily assumed that this

CITY OF NOTTINGHAM.

HEALTH SERVICES.

Preparation for Home Confinement

Midwife .... Tel. No. ....

Address ....

When the Midwife is out a notice on her door will tell you where she may be found.

The **ROOM** in which the birth is to take place should be cleaned a few days before the expected date of confinement. All ornaments, mats and other small articles should be put away, leaving only a minimum amount of furniture in the room. The doctor or midwife will require two tables to be cleared for their use. Washstand or dressing tables may be used in place of the tables.

The **BED** should be made by first placing several thicknesses of newspaper and brown paper over the mattress and covering this with an old clean sheet. Use old, but clean bed linen and nightdresses for the confinement and have a fresh set ready for use afterwards.

[P.T.O.

The following articles will be needed, but you are not expected to go to considerable expense in order to obtain them :—

Midwife :

1 large jug } wash-stand type	Nail brush
1 large bowl } or similar	16 oz. bottle Dettol
1 pint jug	1 lb. cotton wool
2 pint basins	2 clean 1 lb. jam jars
Bedroom slop-pail	

A maternity outfit—to be obtained from your midwife.
Two pairs of sheets, plenty of old linen which has been well boiled and ironed ; it is convenient to keep these in a clean pillowcase.
Kettle and large saucepan, both 4 pint size, and means of heating them.

Mother :

Nightdress	Soap
Nursing brassiere	2 bath towels
2 doz. sanitary towels	2 hand towels
Belt or tape	Face flannel
Chamber or bedpan	

Baby :

3 warm nightgowns	Baby bath or large bowl
3 woollen vests	Plain white soap
Matinee coats and bootees	Baby powder
Napkins	Safety pins
Crepe bandage—3 in. wide	Vaseline
Towel, needle and cotton	

Cot with mattress. This should be got ready with cot sheets and blankets.

IMPORTANT :—No member of the household suffering from cold, skin eruptions or other infectious condition must on any account visit the mother and baby for at least 14 days after the birth.

Relief Midwife :

Name .... Tel. No. ....

Address ....

Figure 4.3 The *Preparations for Home Confinement* list given to women when they booked with a district midwife for a home delivery.

role would be undertaken by the husband. Working-class men usually had two weeks set holiday a year. The pits closed for two weeks in the summer, as did the factories; thus many men had little means of ensuring that they could be with their wives in labour – supposing they wished to be. In the early part of the study this was still very much a society in which men worked in the world and women in the home and such activities as assisting or supporting at birth were still an anathema to many working men.

Thus it was that women needed to choose their supporter. It was often their mother or grandmother, sometimes their sister or mother-in-law and sometimes a friend or neighbour. Newson and Newson reported that 43% of women in their study who had home births had a relative or neighbour in attendance in the room at the moment of birth, while none of the women in the hospital group had anyone they knew with them. They described non-medical helpers at home births as fairly evenly divided into three groups: close female friends, husbands and neighbours. They also stated that there was a helper at every home birth although more than half left the room before the delivery took place (Newson and Newson 1963: 28–9). Those who were asked to support a woman at birth felt very privileged. It was an awe-inspiring task to be assisting the midwife, running upstairs with hot water and cups of tea, and a heart-warming moment when the baby was born.

One of the midwives had this to say:

> Having an experienced woman helping made a lot of difference ... some could just be a nuisance ... wanting to do everything and asking questions ... some just sat downstairs ... others were more like assistants ... they knew what to do and had things ready ... they didn't overstep the mark ... if they were really good you felt confident to let them bath the baby ... sometimes they stayed at the confinement ... it was up to the mother really ... I know we [district midwives] could be bossy ... it was their house though ... I only got bossy if family or neighbours were getting ... too much [meaning overpowering for the mother] ... as time went by more dads were there ... at the delivery ... they still usually had someone else.

The women who helped at birth were well-versed in the preparations. A large pile of newspapers were collected, some to put into the bed and others to scatter over the floor while the mother was pacing about in labour in case she should bleed or her membranes rupture over the linoleum or the midwife spill lotion on the floor. Cotton sheets were passed from house to house to be used at delivery and then boiled for the next confinement; old sheets were torn into strips to be used as drawer sheets and some hemmed as cot sheets. One month before the baby was due she would be told to put a rubber sheet in the bed in case her 'waters broke'. Every day towards the end of the pregnancy a hot-water bottle was put into the cot, to keep it aired.

Supporters knew how to make the delivery bed: a rubber sheet went on the mattress, a boiled cotton sheet went on top, followed by thick layers of newspaper or brown paper between folds of torn sheet, on top of which a drawer sheet would be placed. Once in advanced labour, the mid-wife would open the pack and place the tarred paper and accouchement sheet into the bed. At delivery, blood and liquor would be absorbed into these thicknesses of protection and, as the cleaning-up process took place, layer after layer would be stripped away until the newly delivered woman was left in a clean bed with a clean drawer sheet.

Women knew about fetching the delivery pack after the 32nd week from the midwives' clinic (see illustration below), that it had to remain unopened to preserve sterility and kept out of the reach of children. They knew about buying a pound roll of cotton wool and wrapping it in a nappy to act as a back support to prevent babies from rolling over. It was well understood that there should be an open fire in the house where the placenta could be burned and that the fire needed to be kept in day and night to keep the house warm for the new baby. They knew about the need for a large nursery fireguard firmly attached to the wall. It protected toddlers from the fire and acted as a clothes horse on which to warm the babies' clothes and the midwives' towel and it was in front of this fire that the midwife bathed and the mother fed the baby (see

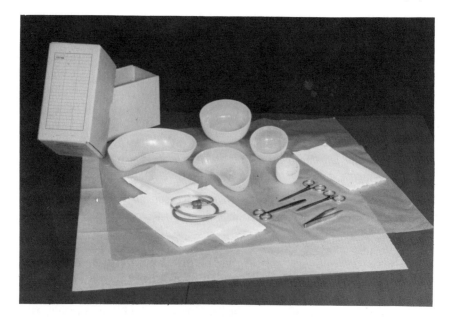

Figure 4.4 The contents of a sterile delivery pack (1964).

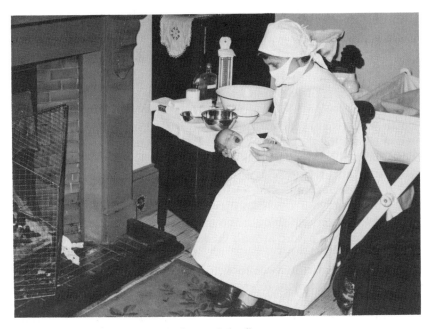

Figure 4.5 Midwife and baby, in front of the fire.

illustration above). Even with all the preparation sometimes things did go wrong.

Annie recalled this incident as a district pupil:

I was doing a home confinement with a midwife ... supervising me ... the delivery was going fine ... the head was just about crowning ... when the money went in the meter ... panic no one had got any pennies ... unforgivable really ... as it was one of the things they were warned about ... anyway ... the grandmother nipped down and lit a candle ... I was still doing the delivery in the dark ... trying to reassure the mother ... the grandmother put the candle at the side of the bed ... as I leaned over my apron brushed over it ... and caught light ... and set my dress alight ... Miss Hughes [the midwife] ... was very calm and said, 'Remember your patient' ... as she batted the flames with her bare hands ... the grandmother was crying ... the mother was busy ... and by this time the baby was born ... by now I could see what I was doing as my dress was lighting up the room ... Miss Hughes said hang on to the baby ... which fortunately was crying its head off ... Miss Hughes had managed to put the flames out ... my clothing burned down to my knickers and bra at the back ... Miss Hughes burned her hands dousing the flames ...

after we had cleared up and made sure mum and baby were alright we went outside and I saw how badly the midwife's hands were burnt ... she said 'come along I'll drive you to the hospital' ... we both had treatment and came back on duty ... I went to the linen room to get another dress ... the linen room lady said, 'You must take better care of your uniforms, they don't grow on trees'.

Women were given a one-off payment, the maternity grant, intended to assist in off-setting the cost of birth: in 1953 the grant was £4 (Carter and Dodds 1953: 612). Most women knew that the only real extra expense for home birth was the cost of heating in the winter. A jam jar with cotton wool in the bottom containing a solution of dettol could be used to store the thermometer, and bowls and jugs from around the house could be cleaned and set on one side for the midwife to use. The baby bath and carry cot would be passed around the neighbourhood.

At the home assessment visit, in addition to looking at the home conditions the district midwife looked at the layout of the room in which the birth would take place to ensure it was possible for her to get access to the woman as she lay in bed, that the bed was a working height and that the woman would not disappear in the middle of a sagging mattress in labour. Home birth almost invariably took place in the main bedroom in the double bed in which the couple usually slept. The midwife took for granted that immediately after the delivery the husband would return to the bed to sleep with his wife.

Audrey recalled this incident:

I was called at 8 in the morning to a labour ... she was getting on ... she'd called the neighbour and got back in bed beside her husband ... he'd only just got in bed after being on nights ... a taxi driver ... she didn't want to disturb his sleep before she had to ... By the time I arrived she was pushing ... I delivered the baby with her husband in bed ... he'd woken up by then, but felt too daft to get out in his pyjamas.

District midwives were generally not prescriptive about labour, they gave general advice about having a warm bath (if the woman had access to a bathroom). They gave advice about eating in labour based on their own experience. Any woman who became at risk of a general anaesthetic would be starved immediately, but otherwise women would be encouraged to eat if they wanted to, but discouraged from eating heavy meals or anything slow to digest. They were persuaded to drink well in labour.

Women did not usually put themselves to bed when labour began, unless it was the middle of the night when they would often stay in bed to avoid disturbing the whole household. During the day they tended to go about their daily chores, get the children off to school, go to the corner

Newfield Road
Sherwood,
Notts.

November 18th 1956.

Dear Nurse Tatton,

I've called hoping to see you a few times but, as expected, always found the list on the door! Now I think it's high time you were warned that I'm afraid I'm going to need your help again next (April 25th.) (Last period started July 18th.) That is if you'll give it, please, and

won't already (booked up. Isn't that time of year pretty futile well Babies? At least I'm not likely to find you out in a bog as Master David did.

He seems to be doing very well but he how times as much trouble as Helen ever was, cutting all his teeth with a different complaint. Spoilt, the most angel, I suspect.

I hope you are all well. Richard and Sarah are all well. Seeing you again is about the only bright spot I can found in this to-do. That & the 10/- of course!

Yours sincerely

Figure 4.6 A letter giving insight into the way in which pregnancy and birth were viewed by one mother in 1956.

shop, get the house in order, prepare the evening meal, do the ironing or have a neighbour in for a cup of tea. The helper would be sent for, the cot and bed prepared and plans laid. During this time the midwife would come and go, keeping a regular check on mother and baby. In the case of grande-multips or women with a history of precipitate or difficult labour the midwife would stay with her if possible throughout labour. The woman generally put herself to bed when labour became intense and she needed to concentrate on the job in hand. Most babies were born in the prepared bed, but all the midwives in the study had undertaken home births in an alternative position, sometimes by accident and occasionally by design.

What most women achieved from a home birth was to be confined in a loving environment with people of their choice present. To continue to share the marriage bed after the delivery, so that the couple adjusted to the new baby together in mutual support. That the mother remained as the head of the household, ensuring that the children went to school and the domestic chores were accomplished even if she was in bed. If the midwife's time was scarce, there was always someone to bath the baby and make the bed, but it was the person the woman had chosen who performed the tasks she asked them to do.

Newson and Newson's study showed that many of the babies born at the time of this study were unplanned but the majority were welcomed at delivery. Arguably, being delivered at home lent something to the bonding process which some say is sometimes missing from birth today. The letter on page 83 to Joyce Tarlton gives some insights into the way in which pregnancy and birth were viewed by one of the mothers in 1956.

INSIGHTS FROM THE REGISTERS OF WOMEN 'DELIVERED AT HOME'

At Appendix C an abridged extract from the early 1960s register of one of the city midwives is reproduced giving as much information as possible, while maintaining the anonymity of midwife and mothers. The register was the midwife's contemporaneous record of her deliveries, written at or as soon as possible after the birth. The detailed account of the progress of labour and delivery was made in the midwife's labour notes, which are not shown. Some columns of the register have been excluded, such as name and address of the mother. The date of discharge, the date and time of the midwife's arrival and the time of the infant's birth have also been omitted as they are irrelevant in this discussion. Similarly, the column for drugs used at or shortly after labour has been omitted as the use of drugs is not part of this study.

This midwife gave a short account of delivery, using the remarks column to identify abnormal situations. Other midwives managed to squeeze a synopsis of the labour into this space. The Supervisor of Midwives did not impose a standard form of 'book-keeping', allowing midwives to show their individuality providing the record-keeping was correct, adequate and legible.

This extract shows the range of age, parity and circumstances of a few of the mothers delivered at home. It has already been established that some 52% of mothers most likely did not fulfil the criteria for home birth, so in that respect this excerpt is typical. However, had other pages been chosen they might have shown a twin birth, premature births or flying squad calls. So in that regard there is no such thing as a typical extract.

The age range and parity of the mothers covers nearly 30 years from the 16- and 17-year-old primigravidae to the 45-year-old woman who had had 16 previous pregnancies. These three deliveries give interesting insights into social background. The 45-year-old mother was an example of many, well-known to district midwives, because of the number of times they had cared for them. Typically they would present at booking clinic for confirmation of pregnancy and selection for place of booking. One reason for attending was to obtain a 'Certificate of Expected Confinement' with which to claim their maternity grant. Having been advised that a hospital birth was necessary, they would attend once, to book, and then default on all further appointments. In labour or after delivery the district midwife would be sent for. Such women had no intention of having a hospital birth and for this reason district midwives often preferred to book them for home birth in the first place, believing that a planned home birth was preferable and safer than a planned hospital birth which was never destined to take place. Once booked with the district midwife, she would follow them up at home even if the women were more in awe than appreciation, as one woman who was the reluctant recipient of care in the 1950s described:

> As soon as the midwife's bike appeared, I sent the young one two doors up to fetch the ... cup and saucer. She was the only woman on the road with a matching cup and saucer ... we all borrowed it for visitors ... I would run and wipe the 'lavvy' seat ... I had four boys you see ... the old man would push his paper down his waistcoat and slip over the back fence ... to next door, he was really terrified of the midwife ... I'd be left to face the music.
>
> *(Allison 1989: 7)*

These women had their own reasons for not wanting a hospital birth. Oakley (1984) discussed the issue 'Why don't women attend', and cites the Parsons and Perkins, Nottingham, study of 90 antenatal care attendants (which identified three distinct groups of non-attenders: 'frightened

teenagers', 'competent child bearers' and 'poor obstetric history combined with massive social problems' (Oakley 1984/1986: 271–2). Their
large families were reliant upon them and they would not be willing to
leave them with relatives in their absence. Many had a real fear that their
children would be taken into care and never returned to them. Some had
a complete disdain of the concept of hospital birth, having had so many
pregnancies they felt they knew as much about it as the doctor. Others,
who were socially disadvantaged, felt uncomfortable away from home.
Frequently they had no nice clothes or pretty nightwear, as money, which
was always scarce, was spent on the family. Husbands, if working, were
unable to offer any real assistance and if not working were not always
inclined to assist.

Wedge and Prosser (1973), in their study of 10 504 children born in
1958, demonstrated how social disadvantage pervaded every avenue of
a child's life. The socially disadvantaged were shown to be continually
struggling against the odds; 23% were badly housed, were single parents
or had a large family of children. The Midlands, where Nottingham is
situated, was shown to be among the worst affected areas. Women
availed themselves of less antenatal care and gave birth to children that
were generally smaller in weight who had parents who were more likely
to suffer from apathy, dislike of authority and general lack of interest.
Such parents were more likely to live in high-rise flats, caravans and
maisonettes, to share rooms and beds, and 90% were likely to suffer
from sleep loss. There was, however, no evidence that a poor start in life
and poor family circumstances resulted in parents who cared less about
their offspring than parents who were from a more advantaged background.

The evidence of the midwives' registers and interviews, the number of
women referred for and refused hospital beds on the grounds of poor
social conditions combined with the evidence of Newson and Newson's
study and the Perinatal Mortality Survey (1963) indicate that a large
number of home births in Nottingham occurred to women who were
socially disadvantaged.

The records of the 16- and 17-year-old primigravidae are interesting as
they both booked for care very early in pregnancy and given this, their age
and nulliparous status would almost certainly have chosen home birth.
Hospital birth would have been offered to such young primigravidae who
booked early. Two explanations are likely: first, that they were married
and pleased to be pregnant; second, that they were unmarried and living
at home and had been pressed by their parents to a home birth in order
to keep the matter as quiet as possible. Such births would sometimes take
place at a grandmother's or an aunt's house and the baby taken for adoption from there. On balance it is most likely that these girls were married,
as an unplanned pregnancy would not have been admitted to at such an

early stage in the pregnancy. Where adoption was planned, it was usually recorded in the midwifes' register.

From 14 deliveries we see that 12 were booked for home birth, one was booked for hospital birth and one was not booked nor had she had any antenatal care. While a general practitioner had been booked by 11 of these women, none were present at delivery, although in the case of the unbooked 19-year-old who sustained a macerated stillborn anencephalic birth, a GP was sent for and probably arrived shortly after the birth. Nevertheless, the mother was kept at home and nursed by the district midwife.

Only three of the women booked in early pregnancy: the usual advice at that time was to wait until two 'periods' had been missed and many waited much longer. Indeed, five women booked at or after the seventh month of pregnancy and two less than a month before delivery. Undoubtedly, part of the reason for the delay in booking of some was because they suspected that they would be referred for hospital birth and so left booking until it was too late to be referred.

Three of the women delivered in the 37th or 38th week of pregnancy with babies weighing about 6lb; one was of unknown gestation and another more than 42 weeks.The birthweights of the remainder were average except for the stillborn anencephalic fetus of unknown gestation and the 42-year-old woman, the last record shown, whose baby weighed 10lb 12 oz. All were in a satisfactory condition at discharge.

The reader will be interested that the babies' weights were all recorded in multiples of 4 ounces. This was because the balance scales used by district midwives for full-term babies were only marked in 4-ounce bands; birthweights were rounded up or down to the nearest 4-ounce mark, unlike the scales shown in the photograph on page 88 which are the full scales with measurements in half ounces, used by the premature baby midwives.

Most of the women were within an acceptable age range for home birth, having first, second, third, fourth, fifth or six babies, whose pregnancy and births were uncomplicated. It is very likely that the majority of them, whatever the circumstance, were delivered at home because they chose to be. The area in which they lived mainly comprised back-to-back terraced houses which, during the course of the following ten years, were demolished to be replaced by high-rise flats which in their turn were pulled down 15 years later.

MATERNAL DEATHS TO
CITY OF NOTTINGHAM RESIDENTS

By 1959 the maternal mortality rate had dropped to 0.38 per 1000 births

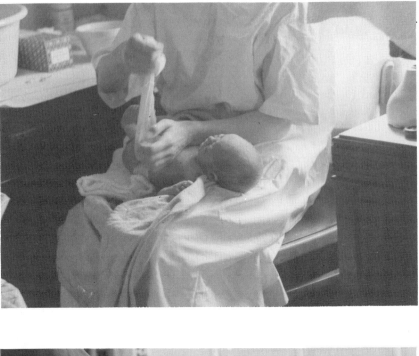

(a)

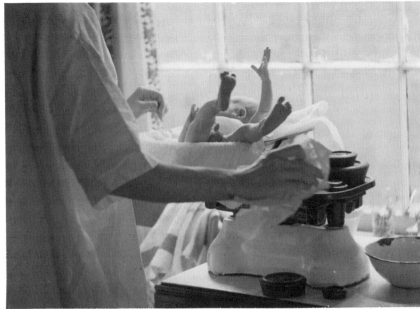

(b)

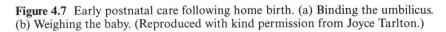

Figure 4.7 Early postnatal care following home birth. (a) Binding the umbilicus. (b) Weighing the baby. (Reproduced with kind permission from Joyce Tarlton.)

in England and Wales, a fall from 0.97 in 1949, and was no longer a useful outcome variable for epidemiological study. However, whenever there is discussion of past systems of maternity care, questions about maternal death arise. The following table is given to illustrate the extent of maternal death in Nottingham during the period when the domiciliary midwifery service was a major provider of midwifery care.

Table 4.1 Maternal death by place of birth: city residents 1949–72

Year	Home MD	Live home birth	Hosp. MD	Live hosp. birth
1949–54	6	15 670	9	15 342
1955–60	0	16 683	27	16 142
1961–66	0	17 416	14	19 578
1967–72	0	9 670	14	22 685
Total	6	59 439	64	73 747

Source: City of Nottingham Medical Officer of Health Reports, Nottingham 1949–72.
MD = maternal death

There were 59 439 home births between 1949 and 1972 with six maternal deaths, all in the period 1949–54. Three were caused by obstetric shock and post-partum haemorrhage, one from uraemia and one from sepsis. The sixth was also caused by obstetric shock but the Medical Officer's report records that she was 'unbooked and unattended, skilled assistance being summoned too late to be of any avail' (City of Nottingham 1953: 26). There is no evidence of any maternal death at home or, apparently, associated with a woman booked for home birth after 1954 until the service was disbanded in 1972. This was confirmed by the Supervisor of Midwives who could recall no incidence of maternal death at home after 1954. There were none among the 11850 births in the registers of the 14 district midwives, which comprise the data for this study.

In the same period there were 73 747 hospital births and 64 maternal deaths. Six were due to obstetric shock, 19 to medical conditions, 10 to pulmonary embolism, 11 to abortion or ectopic pregnancy, two following Caesarean section, three to sepsis, three to toxaemia and the others from causes which were not given in the Medical Officer's Report.

No epidemiological conclusions can be drawn from these data; what is clear, however, is that for whatever reasons district midwives demonstrated the ability to recognize conditions with which they were not qualified to deal. Despite the fact that they were required to deliver many women at home who now might not be considered safe for home birth, after 1954 they appear to have ensured that women were safe at delivery. This conclusion is supported by the findings of the Wormerveer study of 7980 pregnant women booked consecutively at a practice of free-standing midwives between 1969 and 1983, in The Netherlands. This concluded that selection of pregnant women into groups with high and low risk is possible with the relatively modest means available to the midwife (Van Alten, Eskes and Treffers 1989: 656–62).

STILLBIRTHS TO CITY OF NOTTINGHAM RESIDENTS

Drawn from the Medical Officer of Health Reports, the following table illustrates the number of births, per triennia, occurring at home and hospital to city residents, and the number of stillbirths by place and rate. It shows the swing from home to hospital birth, with more than 50% of births occurring at home in the period 1961 to 1963, reducing to 25% in the period 1970 to 1972.

It demonstrates that while the number of stillbirths occurring at home and hospital declined over time, there was an apparent upward trend in the stillbirth rate for babies born at home at the end of the period, but the difference was no greater than is compatible with chance variation. Nevertheless, data such as this was used to support the argument that all birth should take place in hospital, on the grounds that babies delivered at home were born to a carefully selected group of low-risk mothers living in suitable social conditions who could thus expect a near zero stillbirth and perinatal death rate. As discussed previously, this was not the case.

Table 4.2 Live births and stillbirths to city residents by place of birth: 1955–72

Year	Live births		Stillbirths		Stillbirth rate	
	Home	Hospital	Home	Hospital	Home	Hospital
1955–57	8011	7770	87	269	10.9	34.6
1958–60	8672	8372	66	286	7.6	34.1
1961–63	9354	9172	59	285	6.1	31.0
1964–66	8062	10 406	39	297	5.2	28.5
1967–69	5987	11 409	32	242	5.3	21.2
1970–72	3682	11 162	23	181	6.2	16.2
Total	43 768	58 291	306	1560	6.9	27.6

Source: City of Nottingham Medical Officer of Health Reports 1955–72.

Using data from the personal registers of 14 district midwives, it is possible to give more insight into the background of some of the stillbirths which occurred at home. Fifty-six (18.3%) of the 306 stillbirths shown above have been identified from the registers. The number of stillbirths identified in the registers indicates that they are a representative sample in terms of numbers, as the registers contain details of 19% of home births in the period. The following table offers a more detailed analysis.

Table 4.3 Fifty-six stillbirths attended at home by city midwives 1955–72

Year	Home booked	Hospital booked	Unbkd	GP booked	% Not bkd for home	Total
1955–63	17	1	6	3	37	27
1964–72	9	10	8	2	69	29
Total	26	11	14	5		56

Source: Personal registers of 14 City of Nottingham district midwives.

The table shows the stillbirths subdivided into two eight-year periods: 1955 to 1963 (the last year in which the number of home births exceeded the number of hospital births in Nottingham) and 1964 to 1972. Twenty-seven stillbirths occurred in the first period and 29 in the second. Twenty-six of the women in the two groups were booked for home birth and 30 were unbooked, booked at hospital, or booked only with the GP, who had made no provision for birth either at home or hospital, nor had he informed the midwife of the woman's pregnancy.

An interesting feature of this data is that of the women in this sample, who sustained a stillbirth at home in the period 1955–63, 37% were not booked for home birth, whereas in the period 1964–72, 69% were not booked for home birth. If the data for 1970–72 is examined separately, it shows that 75% of women in the sample were not booked for home birth. These data support the evidence presented in Chapter 3 about the number of women who were hospital booked or unbooked but delivered at home.

This story was told to me by Olga in a letter in 1991:

Mrs H ... attended a night labour call. Having assessed the woman she was unable to hear the fetal heart. She informed the woman's husband and told him that she was going out to call an ambulance. The husband went berserk, ran outside and fetched a rope, with which he attempted to hang Mrs H ... from the banister. However, she was very petite and fit and quickly jumped over the banister and ran out of the house. She called an ambulance and the police. It transpired that the father had a long history of mental illness and he was last seen being transported to the local mental hospital by several burly policemen.

Although it was not possible to retrieve Tilly's registers (they were probably lost in the Perth Street flood, see page xv) she had this to say about her experience of stillbirth as a district midwife during the period 1959–66;

My busiest year was 1965 when I had 107 deliveries ... I had 720 deliveries altogether ... there were two stillbirths among them ...

One was a gravida four who developed anaemia of pregnancy and then I diagnosed an IUFD [intra-uterine fetal death] ... but she didn't want to go into hospital ... so I delivered her at home ... The other was a gravida eight, Jamaican lady who booked at the end of her pregnancy ... when I arrived at the house she was well advanced in labour ... at delivery the baby was unresuscitable ... Despite these sad times working on the district was my happiest working experience.

Another midwife whose registers are now lost had this to say about her short time on the district:

I loved it [working as a district midwife] ... I think I had about 300 deliveries ... I was lucky, none of my booked patients had stillbirths ... but I had three altogether ... all women who hadn't booked at all ... Two were young girls ... one was a prostitute.

It is evident from this and the information on page 95 related to BBAs that stillbirth at home, over the whole period, was more often associated with hospital and unbooked women than to those booked for home birth.

RESUSCITATION OF NEW-BORN

In 1958 Nottingham's district midwives were issued with 'Sparklets' oxygen apparatus; this, together with Vandid, was the method of resuscitation of the new-born available to city midwives. Over the following ten years, a record was kept of the number of babies to whom oxygen was administered at birth. The table illustrates that as the stillbirth rate

Table 4.4 Home births and oxygen administration: 1958–67

Year	Number home births	Babies given oxygen	Percentage
1958	2863	64	2.2
1959	2933	65	2.2
1960	2876	31	1.1
1961	2858	28	1.0
1962	3323	24	0.7
1963	3173	20	0.6
1964	2969	17	0.6
1965	2596	19	0.7
1966	2497	14	0.6
1967	2216	11	0.5
Total	28 304	293	1.0

Source: City of Nottingham Medical Officer of Health Reports 1958–67.

declined over the years, so did the percentage of babies to whom oxygen was given at birth. This implies that these experienced midwives saw little advantage in the routine administration of oxygen at birth in terms of reducing the incidence of stillbirth. When Audrey was asked about this she said, 'I used it regularly ... twice a year in the back garden ... to test it was working.'

From oral evidence it appears that midwives used oxygen with enthusiasm when it was first issued but soon came to the conclusion that it was unnecessary in the majority of cases; experience taught them which babies were severely compromised and in need of oxygen. In 1958 the number of stillbirths to home deliveries in Nottingham was 28; the number of babies to whom oxygen was administered was 64; while in 1967 there were nine stillbirths and oxygen was administered to only 11. No scientific conclusions can be drawn from these data but it appears to be an interesting example of how midwives developed practice from experience.

UNATTENDED BIRTHS (BORN BEFORE ARRIVAL OF MIDWIFE (BBAs) TO CITY RESIDENTS 1956–72

The personal registers of the City of Nottingham district midwives have been scrutinized for all incidence of BBAs between 1956 and 1972. Registers for the earlier period have not been used as they were different in format and did not contain sufficient relevant information. Deliveries counted as BBAs were those where the baby was entirely delivered before the arrival of the midwife. In such cases this was clearly noted in the register, which would have no description of the labour or of the presentation of the baby. In contrast, a birth which was actually occurring as the midwife arrived would not be described as a BBA: she would witness both the presentation and the birth and would be able to record with confidence a vertex or breech delivery and the condition of the baby at the moment of birth. The clear distinction, in record-keeping terms, between attended and unattended births has obvious implications in possible cases of litigation.

There were 41 248 home births in Nottingham during the period 1956–72. The midwives in the study undertook and recorded 8794 (21.0%) of those births, of which 443 (5.0%) were BBAs, 329 to women booked for home birth, 66 to women booked to deliver in hospital and 49 to women who had had no antenatal care nor booked a place of birth. The number of women in this data who were unbooked or hospital booked (115) and sustained a BBA gives further support to the elaborated chart on page 70 showing the likely extent of change of place of birth in labour. Translated as a percentage of all home births in the study, the number of hospital and unbooked women who were likely to have sustained a BBA over the whole period was 747, in addition to those where the midwife arrived during the course of labour or at delivery.

Women booked for home birth usually had a BBA because of precipitate labour, although it is possible to see, from their registers, that the midwives were often attending another birth at the time a BBA occurred. Women booked for hospital birth or unbooked, who had BBAs at home, were attended by a district midwife who registered the birth as a home birth.

Despite delivering at home, these 443 women are far from a straightforward selection in the 'low risk' category. Selection for place of birth using criteria related to age, parity, maturity of pregnancy, obstetric, medical and family history was complicated by many factors, including gestation at booking and social class (see Chapter Two). In deciding to what extent these women were suitable for home birth the contemporary criteria described on page 43, and below, will be applied as far as possible:

- As far as can be ascertained the women's general physical state is unimpaired.
- She is pregnant for the second, third or fourth time, the previous pregnancies, labour and puerperia having been normal and she is under 35 years of age or, if a primipara, she is under 30 years of age.
- She is known to have no Rhesus antibodies.
- The home conditions are suitable.
- In addition and in keeping with local policy, women who went into labour before 36 weeks gestation and those who were more than 42 weeks gestation are counted as outside the criteria for home birth, as are girls under 16 years of age (see page 44).

The registers do not necessarily give all this information. Records routinely include age, parity and maturity of pregnancy; where midwives wrote additional information, such as 'diabetic mother', it has been included. However, there is no insight into the height, stature, weight or haemoglobin levels of these women. Thus the number of women shown in this table to have fallen outside the criteria for home birth is less than would have been the real case.

Table 4.5 Women experiencing BBA by those who fell outside criteria for home birth: 1956–72

	Total	Outside	Percentage
BBAs booked for home birth	328	173	53
BBAs booked for hospital birth	66	44	67
Unbooked BBAs	49	38	78
Total	443	255	58

Source: City of Nottingham district midwives' personal registers.

Fifty-eight per cent of all women having BBAs fell outside the criteria for a home birth, including 53% of those booked for home, 67% of those booked for hospital and 78% of the unbooked.

Some women in all categories had more than one factor which contraindicated a home birth.Among them were 15- and 16-year-old primigravidae with premature labours, a 38-year-old gravida 15 premature birth, a 36-year-old gravida 7 pre-term twin birth. In addition, a 34-year primigravida with known heart disease being treated for ascites (presumably the pregnancy), whose pregnancy had gone undiagnosed, spontaneously delivered a 6lb 12oz baby at home, sustaining a third-degree tear.The child fell to the floor and the cord snapped. The woman was not transferred to hospital and mother and baby were successfully nursed at home by the district midwife.

MATERNAL AND PERINATAL OUTCOMES

There was no maternal death in the study of BBA's, whether home, hospital or unbooked for care. The perinatal death rate, over the whole period in this sample of 443 women, was 29 per 1000 births. It could be argued that this high death rate was the consequence of unattended birth. However, when the perinatal death rates are compared according to intended place of birth, a different picture emerges.

Table 4.6 Perinatal death by place of booking: 1956–72

Intended place of birth	Number BBAs	Births	Perinatal deaths	PNMR
Home	328	328	1	3.0
Hospital	66	67*	5	75.0
Unbooked	49	52*	7	142.0
Total	443	447	13	29.0

*Includes some twin births. Source: District midwives' registers.

The perinatal death rate in the home-booked group was 3.0 per 1000 births, despite the fact that almost as many booked for home fell outside home-birth criteria, as did those booked for hospital. It is evident that a higher proportion of women who were hospital booked or unbooked had a BBA following premature labour or intrauterine fetal death.

The hospital-booked group had a perinatal death rate of 75.0 per 1000 births. Some difference between the home and hospital groups is accounted for by the slightly higher number of women who had contraindications to home birth. However, this alone could not account for the much higher mortality rate of hospital-booked women.

The unbooked women had the highest percentage who fell outside the criteria for home birth and the highest perinatal death rate at 142 per 1000 births. The difference in the percentage of women in each group who fell outside home-birth criteria does not explain the huge differences in perinatal death. The wide outcome variation for perinatal death between intended place of birth reflects those of Campbell *et al.* in their study (Campbell *et al.* 1984: 721). One way of further examining the likely explanation is to consider the cause or circumstances of these 13 deaths.

Table 4.7 Cause/circumstances of perinatal death in 13 women who had BBAs: 1956–72

Intended place	Age	Parity	Gestation in weeks	Cause/circumstance of BBA from registers
1. home	32	6	36	5lb 2oz baby xferred to SCU, died 4th day. ? Cause
2. hospital	20	Primipara	?	Stillborn anencephalic infant
3. hospital	24	3	43	Macerated stillbirth 6lb 7 oz
4. hospital	30	Primipara	30	Macerated stillbirth 11lb 5oz
5. hospital	20	3	?	Macerated stillbirth 2lb
6. hospital	19	Primipara	28	Stillbirth 3lb 4oz, quick labour
7. unbkd	25	2	30	Stillbirth, no details
8. unbkd	22	?	32	Stillbirth, no details
9. unbkd	27	4	36	Twins, both BBA. Twin one 6lb 4oz alive. Twin 2 5lb 8oz, dead on arrival of midwife. ? Cause
10. unbkd	16	Primipara	?	Stillbirth 3lb 14oz
11. unbkd	28	3	30	Stillbirth 3lb 6oz
12. unbkd	27	2	40	Stillbirth mw not called until 10 hours after birth. 8lb 12oz
13. unbkd	?	6	28	Stillbirth, no details

Source: District midwives' personal registers.

In addition to stillbirths to hospital and unbooked women, there may have been deaths in the first week of life, of live babies transferred to hospital about which the midwife had no knowledge. Indeed, it is evident from Table 4.7 that no deaths in the first week of life are recorded among the hospital and unbooked women. These mothers and babies were seldom transferred back to the care of the district midwife, unless they took their own discharge from hospital. Thus perinatal deaths for hospital and unbooked women could have been greater than shown.

In the case of home-booked BBAs, women and babies transferred to hospital were always transferred back to the district midwife, who would record perinatal deaths occurring in hospital. These would have been attributed to home-birth data by the Medical Officer of Health.

This data, though limited, demonstrates the likely extent of the number of births which took place at home, but were hospital booked or unbooked. Counted in home-birth statistics, these women were at a hugely increased risk of perinatal death. These findings further elaborate the information in Chapter Three.

MULTIPLE BIRTHS ATTENDED BY DISTRICT MIDWIVES

From January 1955 to December 1967, the Medical Officer of Health kept separate data on multiple births; some of the pregnancies were diagnosed as multiple and others were undiagnosed until labour. During these 13 years, 36 315 births occurred at home, of which 190 were multiple births, 189 were twin deliveries and there was one set of triplets. A general practitioner was reported to have been present at 19 cases. One hundred and seventy twin births and the triplets were delivered or attended following the birth by a district midwife with apparently no doctor in attendance.

No outcomes are given in the reports. Twenty multiple births, where the midwife was in attendance at the birth, have been identified from the personal registers of the midwives in the study who worked at some time during 1955–67.

Table 4.8 Multiple births, attended at delivery by district midwives: City of Nottingham 1955–67

Age	Parity at bking	Place bkd	Gestation in weeks	Twin 1	Twin 2	Twin 1 wght	Twin 2 wght	Xferd to hosp. twin 1	Xferd to hosp. twin 2
25	0	Home	40	Live	Live	5lb 6	6.0lb	No	No
26	1	Home	36	Live	Live	6.0lb	5lb 12	No	No
26	1	Home	42+	Live	Live	5lb 12	6lb 12	No	No
31	3	Hosp.	40+	Live	Live	5lb 4	6lb 0	No	No
29	3	Home	38	Live	Live	6lb 0	5lb 12	No	No
27	2	Home	40	Live	Live	5lb 12	5lb 8	No	Yes
24	2	Home	41	Live	Live	7lb 0	6lb 2	No	No
38	2	Home	36	Live	Live	5lb 12	5lb 0	No	No
37	2	Home	38	Live	Live	4lb 12	5lb 4	Yes	No
21	2	Home	38	Live	Live	6lb 14	4lb 14	No	No
28	3	Home	37	Live	Live	5lb 14	6lb 2	No	No
34	2	Home	41+	sb*	sb*	4lb 0	4lb 0	No	No
21	0	Home	36	Live	Live	4lb 0	3lb 9	Yes	Yes
34	10	Not bkd	34	Live	Live	5lb 5	6lb 4	Yes	Yes
33	2	Home	37	Live	Live	5lb 8	5lb 15	No	No
32	2	Home	36	Live	Live	4lb 13	5lb 7	No	No
27	4	Home	42	Live	Live	6lb 14	5lb 14	No	No
27	3	Home	36	Live	Live	5lb 4	5lb 0	No	No
28	2	Home	38	Live	Live	4lb 12	5lb 7	No	No
21	4	Home	37	Live	Live	5lb 1	5lb 0	No	No

Source: District midwives' personal registers.
*sb = stillbirth

This sample of 20 is too small to draw any conclusions. However, it gives some interesting insights which illustrates other aspects of the study.

In regard to selection and criteria for home birth, these women are an interesting group. In addition to their multiple pregnancy status, a number had other contraindicating factors for home birth today:

- two were primigravida;
- three were grande-multiparae;
- two were over 35 years of age;
- two were 42 weeks gestation;
- one unbooked, 34 week, gravida 11.

These data amplify the findings in Chapter 3 regarding the number of women who fell outside the criteria for a home birth, but were delivered at home.

In regard to infant mortality, one post-mature set of twins was still-born. The mother had been referred for obstetric opinion because of post-maturity and hypertension, having been previously referred for hypertension in early pregnancy and returned to the care of the midwife. The consultant obstetrician performed a surgical induction at home; both twins were stillborn, the second was hydrocephalic. It is not possible to say how this incident came about. However, it is likely that because of the shortage of hospital beds, the induction was undertaken at home because the intrauterine fetal death of both twins had already been diagnosed. The stillbirths were thus attributed to home birth and not to hospital statistics.

The following section deals with the issue of the management of low birthweight babies at home; this sample of multiple births occurring at home gives insight to some of the babies who received care from the premature baby midwives.

Of the 40 babies in this sample, 38 were born alive, 21 weighing 5lb 8oz or more, two of which were transferred to hospital. Nineteen babies weighed less than 5lb 8oz, of which four were transferred to hospital. Two were not booked for home birth; of the four booked for home birth and transferred, two were born to a 36-week gestation 21-year-old primigravida and one to a 37-year-old gravida three. The two stillborn babies were not transferred and were buried from the parents' home. Thus, despite referral to an obstetrician, they were at no time included in hospital birth data.

It is clear that judgement and selection took place about these low birthweight babies about which should be transferred to hospital, where it was believed their chance of survival would be enhanced. This is demonstrated in the home-booked group by the fact that while one twin weighing 5lb 8oz was transferred to hospital, three weighing less than 5lb were not. It is possible that some of the babies transferred to hospital

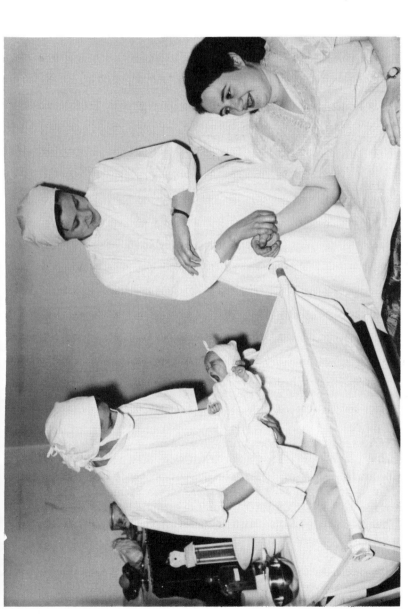

Figure 4.8 A newly delivered Nottingham mother looks on as premature baby midwife and pupil midwife care for her low birthweight baby.

subsequently died, in which case their death, whether in the perinatal, neonatal or infant-mortality group would have been attributed to home-birth data.

MANAGEMENT OF LOW BIRTHWEIGHT BABIES BORN AT HOME

Between 1952 and 1966 there were 85 027 births to City of Nottingham residents, of which 43 173 occurred in hospital and 41 854 at home. Of those 85 027 births, 6586 resulted in babies weighing less than 5lb 8oz, 2051 at home and 4535 in hospital (see multiple births above). Those delivered at home were cared for by the premature baby midwives. The illustration on page 99 shows a young Nottingham mother looking on as the premature baby midwife teaches her to care for her small baby.

Table 4.9 Mortality (28 days) of low birthweight babies, Nottingham 1952–66, by place of birth

Weight	Born at home	Xferd to hosp.	Died	%	Nursed at home	Died	%	Born	Died at hosp.	%
Up to 3lb 4 oz	115	94	51	54.3	21	15	71.4	641	455	71.0
3lb 5oz–4lb 6oz	268	219	34	15.5	49	3	6.1	937	162	17.3
4lb 7oz–4lb 15oz	378	106	16	16.0	272	4	1.5	931	70	7.5
5lb 0oz–5lb 8oz	1290	103	27	26.2	1187	27	2.3	2026	91	4.5
Total	2051	522	128	24.5	1529	49	3.2	4535	778	17.2

Source: Medical Officer of Health Reports 1952–66.

Low birthweight babies born at home were not necessarily booked for home birth, nor if booked for home birth were they necessarily suitable for home birth. Some of those who feature in the home births were booked for hospital but failed to get there either because of precipitate labour or the woman's intention of avoiding hospital birth. The low birth-weight babies born at home also include unexpected home births to women who had concealed their pregnancy and who only summoned aid when the birth was in progress.

Some babies born in hospital had been booked for home birth but transferred either antenatally or in labour when a premature labour or growth-retarded infant was anticipated. Babies of all weights appear to have survived at a similar rate whether delivered at home or in hospital; this reflects the findings of Marjorie Tew (Tew 1995: 249).

The inevitable question arises: why did small babies appear to have a similar chance of survival if born at home, especially since many of their families were from social class five? One plausible hypothesis is lack of stress. Unlike those born in hospital, who were separated from their mother, and nursed in a brightly lit area by a number of different staff, babies born at home were nursed by their mother, with the family's love and support and the midwife's encouragement. This gave the mothers a sense of ownership and control and allowed for early bonding (see Figure 1.8).

Many of the arguments which apply to these local data have already been made by Marjorie Tew (1995) in the context of the Registrar General's statistics. However, what becomes much clearer from this study is the extent to which low birthweight babies born at home were **not** a sample of carefully selected babies, born to low-risk mothers in good social conditions. Past arguments about the outcome of low birthweight babies born at home or hospital have been made on the assumption that women booked for home birth were 'low risk' and that hospital-birth outcomes were alone in being contaminated by the number of babies transferred in. No account has been taken of the fact that home-birth statistics were similarly skewed by the number of unbooked and hospital women delivered at home (see Chapter 3).

Tew (1986: 659–74) postulates that the decline in perinatal mortality has been due to the improvement in maternal health status over time, and suggests that perinatal mortality was higher in hospital because of intranatal interventions. On the face of it, non-interventionist antenatal and intranatal care from a district midwife, coupled with the facilitative and supportive approach from one premature baby midwife in the post-natal period, seems to have had as much success in terms of perinatal mortality as the more medically oriented approach in hospital. Campbell et al. have made similar observations using more contemporary data (1987, 1994).

BREAST-FEEDING RATES AMONG HOME BIRTHS

At discharge, midwives recorded the method of feeding for each home birth. Not all were consistent in recording this information. Sometimes, if a midwife did not carry out the postnatal care of her patient because she was on holiday or sick, she failed to check the method of feeding when she completed her register. In the case of these six sets of registers, the midwives had consistently recorded the method of feeding at birth and discharge. These midwives worked on the district for a substantial time during the period 1957–72 and four of them remained as community midwives until at least 1976. For the purposes of this exercise, data has been used through until 1976. It is not possible to begin the analysis any earlier, as information about the method of feeding was not routinely kept in the earlier registers.

Midwives differed in the way in which they recorded the method of feeding. Some simply wrote 'breast-feeding' or 'artificial feeding'; others included more detail such as 'breast-feeding with some complimentary feeds', or 'artificial feeding-NDM'. About half of district midwives recorded the type of artificial milk used. This included:

National Dried Milk (NDM) – withdrawn in the early 1970s
Cow and Gate
SMA
Trufood
Carnation Evaporated Milk (commonly used for low birthweight babies)
Ostermilk

The data comprises all of the births undertaken by these individual midwives, whether the baby was transferred to hospital, cared for by the premature baby midwife or died in the perinatal period, and the number of babies by those who were being breast-fed (whether totally or with complimentary feeds at the date of discharge).

A number of factors need to be taken into account when considering this data. The length of time that a midwife was statutorily required to attend a mother at home following delivery was reduced from 14 days to ten days during the period of the study. However, midwives frequently visited after the minimum visiting date. Thus the best that can be said about the date of discharge is that it would be a minimum of the tenth postnatal day, and a maximum of the 28th day, except in the rare case of premature babies where they may have been nursed at home for longer.

Table 4.10 Percentage of women breast-feeding on discharge as recorded by six city midwives

Year	1957 to 1958	1959 to 1960	1961 to 1962	1963 to 1964	1965 to 1966	1967 to 1968	1969 to 1970	1971 to 1972	1973 to 1974	1975 to 1976
Number of births	535	656	734	800	831	821	678	474	290	96
% B/fding	80	73	66	47	37	26	17	17	23	30

Source: Personal registers of six City of Nottingham district midwives.

These data have no statistical significance in terms of the wider debate about the decrease over time in the incidence of breast-feeding. However, since this historic data has been unearthed it makes an interesting snapshot of the breast-feeding pattern among home-delivered, mainly working-class women over a 20-year period.

Midwives had a very clear duty to vigorously advocate breast-feeding as a preferred choice.

It is expected that the midwife will do her utmost to promote breast-feeding and will encourage patients to prepare their breasts during pregnancy.

(Appendix A: Instructions to Midwives April 1957)

Indeed, it was a requirement of the Central Midwives Board that the attendant midwife should notify the local authority of every woman who intended to artificially feed her baby. The requirement was not abolished until 1969 (CMB 1969).

Breast-feeding rates among this group of women declined over time from a high of 80% of mothers breast-feeding at discharge in 1957–8, when women were nursed until the 14th postnatal day. By 1969–70, when women were only routinely nursed until the 10th postnatal day and were no longer guaranteed continuity of carer, breast-feeding rates at discharge had dropped to 17% among this generally working-class group of women.

In 1959–60 Newson and Newson (HMSO 1974: 45) found that in a sample of Nottingham mothers delivered at home and hospital, 60% were breast-feeding at the end of a fortnight, while 73% of women in this small, exclusively home-delivered group were breast-feeding at or after the 14th postnatal day.

By 1975–6, when the number of home births by these midwives had dropped to 18% of the 1957–8 total, the breast-feeding rate had increased again to 30%. The probable explanation is that the women who delivered at home in 1976 were more likely to be predominately drawn from the articulate middle classes who insisted on home birth, after the opening of the new maternity unit, when the majority of working-class women had been persuaded into hospital.

It is interesting to speculate how these midwives in 1957–8 helped to achieve an 80% overall breast-feeding rate among women who were generally poor and often inadequately nourished. Part of the explanation may lie in the fact that in those years women were guaranteed continuity of care from their own midwife or at worst from her partner, throughout the pregnancy, labour and postnatal period. Indeed, many of them saw no other carer than their midwife. However, it is evident from the midwives' registers that there was a considerable outcome variation between midwives. While midwife two had a breast-feeding rate at discharge of 92% in 1957, midwife one achieved only 73%. Similarly, while midwife six had 40% breast-feeders in 1975, midwife three had only 12%. Because this is such a small sample of the district midwives and it is clear that there are large individual outcome variations between midwives, it is not possible to relate this data to Table 4.11.

A further insight into the possible influence of continuity of carer on the likelihood to breast-feed can be found in some interesting data recorded by the Supervisor of Midwives between 1951 and 1960. From the data collated from the Central Midwives Board, returns of those women who commenced artificial feeding the following table is compiled.

Table 4.11 Number of women intending to artificially feed by place of birth

Year	Hospital births	Artificial feeding	Percentage	Home births	Artificial feeding	Percentage
1951–52	5425	861	16	5029	306	6
1953–54	4761	783	16	5221	315	6
1955–56	5027	1155	23	5167	332	6
1957–58	5342	636	12	5707	445	8
1959–60	5773	777	13	5809	365	6
Total	26 328	4212	16	26 933	1763	6.5

Source: City of Nottingham Medical Officer of Health Reports 1951–60.

The Supervisor of Midwives collated all data related to artificial feeding for home and hospital. This data illustrates that there is a consistently higher number of hospital-delivered women who chose to artificially feed their baby by the date of discharge than home-delivered women. Two explanations come to mind: first, the influence of the individual midwife who gives continuity of care and second, that hospital-delivered women were more likely to have experienced instrumental deliveries which may have left them less inclined to battle with the early inconveniences of breast-feeding.

CONCLUSION

In this chapter there has been an attempt to give context and texture to the mothers and babies who were delivered at home in Nottingham. Something of the home-birth process has been examined and the outcomes from a variety of perspectives have been reviewed.

Evidence on p. 55 shows that for the majority of women booked for home birth it was their first choice. There is some evidence of their satisfaction with the service and no evidence of dissatisfaction; nevertheless, domiciliary midwifery had already been doomed to virtual extinction by the Peel Report (1970). While Nottingham trailed behind the rest of Britain the change was inevitable, although even the most ardent obstetricians acknowledged that the change was not of the mothers' choosing.

> Midwifery is at present shared between consultant obstetric units ... and a dying domiciliary service ... There is little doubt that the majority of mothers are happier at home with their husband and family close at hand. On the other hand, hospital delivery is infinitely safer.
>
> *(Stearn 1968: 390)*

The mothers and babies of Nottingham in the era of this study existed in a culture which viewed home birth as a normal feature of everyday life, as indeed it remains in Holland (Damstra-Wijmenga 1984: 425) The district midwife was as much a part of local society as the doctor or the postman and was generally respected for her professional expertise. Parents, then as now, were afraid of having stillborn or damaged babies; however, in the main they did not see home birth as any more risky than hospital birth. Indeed, from my own experience there was a certain satisfaction in being booked for home birth: arguably it indicated that your pregnancy and labour were expected to be uneventful.

The outcomes of birth at home, given the social, economic and health status of many of the women, was good, both in terms of maternal mortality, stillbirth and the care of low birthweight babies. Indeed, as Tew has argued, yet more might have been achieved for these women if funds had been made available to improve their social and domestic circumstances, rather than making more maternity beds available. Money spent in improving the home and economic status of a family in order to support a home birth improved the environment for the growing child: an investment in the future, if you like.

Burnell, McCarthy, Chamberlain *et al.* (1982) argued that detaining women with poor social circumstances in hospital after birth did not improve the home conditions and that postnatal care at home by community midwives may be suitable for most women. Indeed, let us take that argument one step further. Money spent in bringing a woman, who preferred home birth, to hospital for two days or ten days because her home was unsuitable for birth, was money wasted. On the 11th day the mother and baby returned to a home which, if unsuitable for a home birth, was certainly unsuitable to raise an infant in.

HOME CONFINEMENT:
OUTCOMES AND EXPERIENCES

Key points

- Six maternal deaths occurred at home in Nottingham during the period of the study. None occurred after 1954.
- The number of stillbirths at home and hospital declined at a similar rate until 1969.
- The apparent upward trend in stillbirths at home in the period 1970–2 is accounted for by the fact that 75% of women in the sample who sustained stillbirths at home were not booked for home birth, but were hospital or unbooked.
- The use of oxygen for resuscitation of the new-born declined from 2.2% of births in 1958 to 0.5% in 1967.
- Midwives in the study attended 8794 home births between 1956 and 1972, of which 443 were BBAs, 329 to home-booked women, 66 to hospital-booked and 49 to unbooked women. The perinatal death rate to the home-booked was 3.0 per 1000, to the hospital-booked 75.0 per 1000 and to the unbooked 142 per 1000.
- One hundred and ninety multiple births occurred at home between 1955 and 1967; a GP was present at 19 of these cases.
- In addition to their multiple pregnancy status, many of the women having a multiple birth at home fell outside the criteria for home birth by parity, gestation and maturity of pregnancy.
- Mortality outcomes of babies born at home between 1952 and 1966 were comparable to those born in hospital, despite the fact that many of the babies born at home were not booked for home birth.

Learning the lessons of the past | 5

This book has been about home birth in Nottingham and about the district midwives who delivered 62 444 babies at home between 1948 and 1972. It has also been about the mothers and families of those babies, their experiences, the outcome of those home deliveries and of the mothers' perceptions of the service they received. Key questions emerge from within the wider descriptive framework of the book in the light of today's changing maternity services. As health authorities and trusts seek to find new ways of organizing midwifery care to meet the challenge to offer 'woman-centred care', how, in comparison, did district midwifery work in terms of organization and caseload? Similarly, to what extent could the work of district midwives be described as team midwifery and what level of success was achieved in terms of continuity of carer and choice?

The Winterton Report (HMSO 1991) gave weight to the view that there is no evidence that birth in a consultant-led unit is the safest or most desirable option for all women. It also called for the proper and full utilization of midwives' skills. In the continuing debate about the place of birth and the safety of mothers and babies to deliver anywhere other than a consultant maternity unit, other questions arise. What were the criteria and selection processes for home birth? What were the outcomes of home delivery in terms of the safety of mother and baby and client satisfaction in this sample of births undertaken with almost total midwife-led care?

These questions are now revisited and drawing upon the text, summary conclusions are offered. The study demonstrates that district midwifery services were provided from within discrete, district-based organizations, whose executive and employees all had proven experience and qualification in the field of domiciliary maternity care and public health. There was no financial, functional or executive control from hospital services. However, there was mutual respect and good working relationships between district midwives and obstetricians.

Through most of the period, district midwives carried an average caseload of around 100 cases per annum: almost twice that recommended by the 1949 government working party. This was due to a national shortage of midwives, both on the district and in hospital. Because of the large caseloads, daily workloads were excessive and midwives were 'on call' for 130 hours a week in the early part of the study. However, for six years the district midwives refused an opportunity to reduce their workload and hours by the introduction of a night-rota system because they wanted to attend their own clients in labour.

Undoubtedly, the district midwives of Nottingham were overworked, with too little support and long hours on call. It is the more surprising therefore that in a time of low unemployment, many chose to stay throughout their working life 'on the district'. It is also clear that many district midwives trained with a view to practising in the domiciliary midwifery service. After qualification they entered the service and remained there until they retired.

District midwives did not work in teams but in partnerships. They worked as individual practitioners in a non-hierarchical service, giving caseload care to their own clients and liaising with their partners to ensure reciprocal cover for their clients. They were employed within one of a national network of district-based, non-hospital-allied domiciliary midwifery services which offered home delivery to women across Britain.

District midwives lived within and had responsibility for a geographic 'patch' of the city. Their duties included caring for women booked for home birth and attending all hospital or unbooked women who delivered at home and any emergency, including abortions. In effect, all social and domestic aspects of birth, whether or not it was intended to occur in the home, were the province of the domiciliary midwife.

The district midwives to whom I spoke could see no similarity between what is done today in the name of team midwifery and the way in which they worked. They saw themselves primarily as independent midwives, in the sense that they had their own caseload of women for whom they had total responsibility. They recognized their accountability to the Supervisor of Midwives and their need to offer reciprocal cover to their partner/s to ensure that their own women were cared for by a known carer in their absence.

All district midwives in the study gave continuity of carer throughout the whole childbearing process. In the early period (Phase One) women were assured of being attended in labour by their own midwife or partner, whom they had met in pregnancy. The registers show that midwives mostly delivered their own clients and that some women saw no other carer than their own midwife. In Phase Two, after the night-rota system had been introduced, a woman's chance of having a known carer in labour was still very high but not guaranteed.

There were six maternal deaths at home and 64 in hospital during the period. No maternal deaths seemingly occurred at home after 1954, nor is it apparent that any of those occurring in hospital were attributable to home-booking.

Among other findings it emerges that despite the fact that an estimated 52% of women who were delivered at home in Nottingham did not fulfil the criteria for a home birth, the stillbirth rate for babies born at home was comparable to that of babies born in hospital. Seventy-two per cent of stillborn babies from the registers of the city midwives in the study in the period 1970–72 were not booked for home birth, but were hospital booked or unbooked cases unintentionally delivered at home, counted in home birth statistics. In addition, the low birthweight babies born at home, whether or not it was their chosen place of birth, survived at a similar rate to those born at hospital.

The outcomes for mother and baby were apparently good despite the fact that only 8.6% of women booked for home birth were transferred to hospital care in the antenatal period and 1.1% in or around the time of labour.

Medically led criteria related to obstetric, medical and social conditions grew over time. In 1967 the Ministry of Health issued criteria for normal (home) confinement (see page 43). Nottingham's maternity service was not able to provide sufficient hospital beds for all residents who, according to the criteria, needed hospital birth; therefore some 52% of women who did not fulfil the criteria for a home birth were delivered at home during the life of the local authority domiciliary service.

Selection for place of birth was governed by two factors: first, the criteria for home birth and the availability of beds in hospital. As working-class women tended to book later in their pregnancy, they were less likely to secure a bed. Second, there is evidence of streaming by social class by GPs with a bias to hospital booking among professional and middle-class women who were predominately booked at the only maternity hospital, both for first and subsequent babies.

Although the findings of this study do not present a paradigm for the future provision of maternity services or midwifery care, it is an approach to understanding how one system of care worked in practice and considering whether it offers any notions for the future.

THE 'WHERE TO BE BORN' DEBATE

In their foreword Campbell and Macfarlane (1987) state:

> We are conscious that in focusing on the place of birth we may seem
> to have ignored the question of who provides the care. This reflects

the fact that statistics have been done in a way which tends to make midwives invisible. While they always have and still do attend the majority of births, past arguments have often centred on the position of GPs and obstetricians without taking into account the contribution of midwives and other staff. We are encouraged by the increasing tendency for midwives to do their own research and hope that this will result in fuller information emerging in the future.

This project has been about a small group of district midwives who over a 24-year period delivered some of the 62 444 babies born at home in Nottingham. Except for the occasional presence of a pupil, GP or medical student, they delivered babies single-handedly; indeed, 12 of the 14 midwives in the study said that with the exception of the Supervisor of Midwives they had never had another midwife present at a birth. Two had careers spanning 30 years, each having delivered some 2000 babies at home.

This is one example of the type of care given by district midwives across Britain, offering women the opportunities now being sought in *Changing Childbirth* (HMSO 1993). In Phase One of the study, continuity of carer for women delivered at home or in hospital was mostly achieved, as was the opportunity for women who were delivered at home to have some degree of choice and control in their own environment.

However, this book has not only been about home birth, but about the skills, expertise and knowledge of midwives. The results in the face of poor social conditions and lack of hospital beds demonstrate their decision-making powers, their recognition of cases that were outside their domain and the efficacy of the non-interventionist approach of midwifery care even in difficult cases. This approach to care is no longer confined to domiciliary practice but has been extended through innovation into the hospital maternity-care agenda. Thus this research can be read as evidence of midwife-led care in a time when the obstetric, medical and social-risk factors of many women was arguably far greater than would be the case today.

Two previously unexplored issues which have been the subject of some closely protected beliefs are tested against the available evidence from Nottingham. The assumption that women who were delivered at home were low risk for complication is shown to be flawed. It is probable that 52% of the 62 444 women who had home births in Nottingham during the period of the study did not fulfil the criteria for home birth.

The second assumption is that hospital mortality outcomes were adversely skewed by the number of women transferred to hospital from home. The analysis of data from the midwives' registers and Medical Officer of Health Reports shows that this was not a one-way phenomenon. Home-birth statistics were equally affected by high-risk hospital-booked or unbooked women, who were delivered at home.

This book has been about one system of care, the City of Nottingham domiciliary midwifery service – one of a national network of similar services which for 24 years delivered half of Britain's babies at home.

While half the babies were delivered at home, half were born in hospital. Midwives who gave care in hospital have played little part in this book, because the two services were not integrated at any level. I want to acknowledge the contribution of hospital midwives, for in making 'district midwives' visible there was no intention to make their work anonymous. What became evident while undertaking this research was that in their own way, within the hospitals of the day which were generally smaller, midwives gave a level of continuity of care and carer which would be envied by many today. Indeed, in many hospitals, midwives were essentially the lead carers as there was no resident obstetrician.

Women who were referred to hospital in Phase One had all their care there and were almost guaranteed to be delivered and given postnatal care by someone they had met before. As midwives are now undertaking their own research, it would be good to see an historical study of the organization of pre-Peel hospital maternity services and of the life and work of hospital-based midwives, by a midwife.

There are still midwives in practice who worked in those services and some retired midwives who would remember the immediate era of the implementation of the National Health Service. A number of hospital midwives in Nottingham kept their own birth registers and this was probably not an isolated practice. Many hospital midwives 'lived in' in hospital accommodation for the whole of their working life and gave the same type of dedicated carer service that was given by district midwives. Using hospital archive material and midwives' oral evidence and registers, it should be possible to recreate something of the mood of hospital maternity services of the immediate past and of the work of hospital midwives. Through understanding the past and synthesizing knowledge and experiences in the light of modern developments and consumer wishes, professional maturity and stature grows.

In the 1970s the concept of shared care became normal practice. District midwives were retitled community midwives and became part of the primary health-care team, working with GPs. Home birth was no longer a viable option for most mothers in the drive to hospitalize birth. The role of the geographically based midwife who offered a first point of contact with the maternity service was to fade into history. For some midwives this led to career dissatisfaction; and for some families the virtual annihilation of home birth was the loss of a social and domestic 'rite of passage'.

We must move forward quickly for the next generation of mothers and babies, now that central policy acknowledges the value of midwives' skills. The next important step is to ensure that midwives are ready to take on their role in the future maternity services. Understanding the reality of how district midwives worked helps us to challenge old assumptions and find ways of giving maternity care which is both acceptable to midwives and to women.

Midwives and the future maternity services

In this final chapter, issues arising out of the study are discussed in relation to the role of midwives in today's changing maternity services. Education in preparation for giving 'woman-centred care', our relationship with medical colleagues, concepts of team approaches to midwifery care and caseloads are considered. The grade and status of midwives is also contemplated in relation to the findings of the study.

PAST AND FUTURE EDUCATION OF MIDWIVES

The evidence of this study confirms the belief that midwives in the recent past were well trained for the function they performed. The outcomes of their activities, examined in the light of contemporary scientific knowledge and prevailing economic and social conditions, were good. However, the way in which they were trained and the level of academic qualification they achieved was very different to that of today's midwife.

During Part One training, pupil midwives were taught in schools of midwifery next to the wards in which mothers and babies were given care. In Part Two, they lived and worked 'on the district'. Now student midwives undergo a single period of training within institutions of higher education, far removed from the client. Their time on the community often resembles a ward allocation rather than the experience of yesterday's pupil whose training was transferred to the public health domain and skills into the sociodomestic environment.

During the period of the study, midwife teachers undertook the majority of clinical teaching and assessment. Many had responsibility for

Pupil midwife denotes a learner during the study and student midwife denotes today's learner.

a ward or clinic and their clinical expertise was without challenge. Today, midwife teachers are frequently isolated miles from maternity units and most clinical teaching and assessing is undertaken by clinically based midwives. **In finalizing the move of midwifery education into higher education we must ensure that the clinical expertise of midwife teachers is not lost, for they represent that vital link between theory and practice without which any practically based profession will founder**.

During the study, midwifery curricula were set by the Central Midwives Boards. Part One comprised a grounding in normal and abnormal midwifery and the work of hospital midwives. Part Two concentrated on domiciliary midwifery and in gaining insight into the concept and practicalities of 'public health'. This included the social and domestic responsibilities of district midwives to their clients and the inter-relationship between the well-being of local families and issues of housing, education, social services, sanitation and district nursing and midwifery services. Pupils also learned to be confident and competent enough to undertake home birth. Their training ensured that midwives were ready to practise in any contemporary setting at the point of registration.

At present, midwifery training is a single course, the curriculum is designed by the individual institution and, at the time of writing, validated by the English National Board for Nursing Midwifery and Health Visiting. Despite the fact that as a profession we espouse the importance of relating theory to practice, students are now usually taught the theory away from the clinical setting. Aspects of public health and social care, which are vital components of future strategy to improve maternal and infant mortality and morbidity, are not always reinforced in a way that prepares the student to readily adapt her practice to changing maternity policy.

The separation of education into institutions of higher education has been generally welcomed as a proper recognition of the nature and level of contribution of the caring professions. However, for midwifery it has not been without its difficulties, which were crystallized in a recent report.

> The form of collaborative links for midwifery education has been the result of political negotiations and bargaining where the interests of midwives have sometimes been subsumed under the interests of nursing. As a consequence the midwives' perception of their control over their own education has been weakened.
>
> *(Maggs 1994: 3)*

In addressing the issues of *Changing Childbirth* the role of midwife teacher as theorist and clinician must be clarified, as must ways in which they can offer, with students, continuity of carer to clients. In the report on the newly created pre-registration midwifery education programmes,

Direct but Different, Maggs (1994) made a number of recommendations. Among them were:

- The development of clinical research or joint clinical/teaching activities by midwife teachers and service colleagues would help overcome the separation between service and education.
- In principle and to a large extent in practice, pre-registration midwifery education provides an opportunity for midwives to define more clearly their professional identity as distinct from nurses, to provide a better quality, woman-centred service and to enhance their professional status. It may be seen as part of a professional project to strengthen midwives' claim to a specified occupational territory supported by the credentials of a higher education diploma or degree.

We must take the opportunity now to educate midwives who will give the service required by *Changing Childbirth*. Ways must be found of giving them sufficient experience to gain confidence and competence in normal birth in a variety of settings. There are now midwives, both within the NHS and in independent practice, who regularly practise in this manner and they should be encouraged to take on this role. During the period of the study there was no requirement for all midwives to teach students; those with aptitude, commitment and good practice were singled out for approval as teaching midwives. In this way pupils were assured of a district teacher who was committed to teaching and the best standards of practice were constantly passed down.

In addition to their commitment to teaching pupils, district midwives supervised and taught medical students in the clinical process of home birth. Thus, in addition to the experience of normal childbirth, future doctors were introduced to the reality of the day-to-day lives which many disadvantaged families endured. They were given a first-hand opportunity to witness the interplay between the role of district carers and the public health function of the health department. Similarly, obstetricians taught pupil midwives about the complications of pregnancy and birth both in theory and practice. In this way each had an appreciation of the other's role. Now medical students no longer undertake home birth with community midwives and obstetricians have less involvement in midwifery education as we appear to be severing our ties with our close colleagues. The role of the midwife and obstetrician are interdependent; a successful midwifery service is just as dependent on obstetricians as an obstetric service is upon midwives. The key to a successful relationship between midwives and obstetricians lies in developing a mutual respect and agreement upon each other's role and responsibilities.

The issue of creating an appropriate interface between medical and midwifery education is central to the implementation of a maternity service whose underlying philosophy is 'woman-centred care'. The way ahead educationally must be to strengthen the academic relationship between midwifery and obstetrics, with midwives playing an equal part in the process.

TEAM MIDWIFERY

Over the past decade a variety of new schemes, described as team midwifery, have been introduced. Some are redolent of the philosophy of care once given by district midwives: to take the service to the client rather than always bringing the client to the service. *Mapping Team Midwifery* (Wraight *et al.* 1993) sought to determine the nature and extent of practices being carried out in England and Wales in the name of 'team midwifery'. This study found that few schemes are currently organized in ways which will improve continuity of care (IMS 1993/iii), but did identify a number that could be presented as 'best practice' models.

Early in their report Wraight *et al.* state: 'Maternity care cannot return to the system in operation 50 years ago when continuity of care was simply provided by the woman's own GP and domiciliary midwife' (Wraight *et al.* 1993: 12). This may be so, but no explanation is offered as to why, although at the conclusion of their study they note that team midwifery:

> seems to demand a different style of working for the midwife, for example, flexible and on-call hours and total responsibility for a group of women ... these factors may cause difficulties to the midwife with dependants and to the newly qualified midwife seeking support and advice from her more experienced colleagues.
>
> *(Wraight et al. 1993: 125–6)*

A key feature of midwifery education during the period covered by this project was that in addition to gaining enough experience in both hospital and home settings to ensure competency and confidence to practise in either, pupils had sufficient experience of each type of care to help them decide where they were best suited to practise on qualification. It was well understood that some midwives felt most suited to practise in hospital and others believed they were 'made for the district', just as some doctors choose general practice and some specialize in hospital.

Some would argue that it is as inappropriate to expect a midwife to be able to attend a Caesarean section in the morning and run a community-based antenatal clinic in the afternoon as it is to expect a GP to perform a ventouse extraction occasionally or the obstetrician to come and take morning surgery. Similarly, some would argue that if a midwife's education had given her the whole range of appropriate clinical experience, it would be equally inappropriate to require a midwife to have two years' experience of working in hospital before applying for a community post.

There never has been a time when midwives have provided an equitable nationwide seamless service between hospital and home. There is much to be done in preparing them for the future if the agreement of the 1993 Department of Health consensus conference that 'continuity of care would best be provided by small teams of midwives with their own caseloads working between hospital and community', is to be realized.

Midwives are quick to point out that they are the senior person present at the majority of UK deliveries, that they are the experts in normal birth yet still give midwifery care to all women and babies however complicated the birth may be. These claims are real because at the point of registration midwives are qualified to give the full range of midwifery care, although clinical experience to support the claim that they may undertake care in any setting has been hard to come by in recent years.

New policy makes clear that women should be at the centre of care and while the remit of *Changing Childbirth* did not include social, domestic and economic aspects of care, it was acknowledged that these would be addressed as the practical and philosophical threads of the report were teased out.

Chalmers, Enkin and Keirse (1989) advocated that maternity carers must see childbearing women within their wider social context in order to give them effective care. The 1993/4 Annual Report of the Maternity Alliance indicates that 31.09% of women in Britain in 1994 received a means-tested payment from the Social Fund in comparison to 23.06% in 1989. It is a matter of concern to all maternity carers that almost one-third of Britain's babies are born into relative poverty. Tyler (1994: 552–4) draws attention to the 'inverse care law' in relation to maternity care, arguing that there is a danger that the women who would most benefit from continuity of carer will be the least likely to experience it because the articulate 'middle classes' may, once again, consume the lion's share of the resources.

It is evident from this study that there was a bias to poor families among the women delivered at home between 1948 and 1972. What has emerged shows that these families enjoyed continuity of carer from a midwife who acted as a social support, a role model and a continuing line of reference and ensured that good maternal and infant outcomes were achieved. Indeed, it would not be difficult to argue that the influence of the district midwife had a long-term effect in improving the social and domestic skills of the mothers and that their contribution was a major factor in the general improvement in standards of public health until the 1960s.

Clearly, arguments are arising that not all midwives wish or feel comfortable with the 'new' way of working. Some are happy and giving their best service in the hospital setting, working with obstetricians for women with complicated pregnancies. For those who choose this type of care, these midwives will provide the core of midwifery expertise which remains hospital based.

On the other hand, many midwives are fulfilled and giving best service in a community-based setting, which crosses the home/hospital divide. These midwives will most influence women whose real threats are the long-term consequences of poverty. Community-based midwives are best placed to bring together a package of services to assist pregnant women whose problems may include malnutrition, an inability to access social service resources, smoking, alcohol and drug abuse, non-attendance for care, premature labour, a tendency to unattended birth, a lack of partner or social support, homelessness, illiteracy, itinerancy and mental and physical illness. These midwives are more likely to be working in liaison with general practitioners and other community-based carers.

In putting women and their families at the centre of care, the recommendations of *Changing Childbirth* will greatly assist those who struggle to mitigate the short- and long-term affects of poverty on the women and babies of Britain. However, we must ensure that midwives are facilitiated to give care within a model which best utilizes their skills and fits their choice of care-giving and work pattern, while bringing the most benefit to society. **Choice, continuity and control in their domestic and professional environment must work for midwives as well as for women**.

One of the reasons that the domiciliary service of 1948–72 worked well and produced good outcomes in terms of safety and satisfaction was that district midwives were working where they chose to work. For many, working as a 'district midwife' was a vocation. Similarly, many of the midwives who worked in hospital were professionally fulfilled in that environment. Today it is possible for midwives to work across the hospital/community barrier and give women community-based care and hospital birth: probably the first choice for most women. The key feature of a successful future service will be a dedicated work-force of midwives; indeed, they will be the element by which any changes succeed or fail.

CASELOADS AND WORKLOADS

One way of achieving the kind of care that women want is for midwives to carry their own caseload. However, the lesson that could be learned from this study is that caseloads must be realistic and regularly monitored, with an adequate back-up and relief service.

Once again it may be appropriate for national guidelines to be set with regard to caseloads. The issue of what constitutes an appropriate caseload and workload is influenced by many factors, including:

- number of midwives in partnership/team;
- mix of home- or hospital-booked clients;
- criteria for booking with caseload midwife;
- integrated (seamless) service or separate community/hospital services;
- ratio of clients with special needs;
- geographical spread of clients;
- flexibility of midwives' working hours;
- commitment of midwives to the service;
- location of midwives' base;
- ratio of learners;
- midwives ability to suture perinea;
- communication system;
- relief arrangements/rota system;
- number of midwives attending each birth;
- midwives' other duties, e.g. postnatal care of hospital-delivered women;
- number of cross-boundary referrals;
- transitional care of low birthweight babies;
- level of support workers;
- locus of supervision;
- arrangements for screening tests;
- whether midwives continue with care if women transferred to consultant care;
- transport;
- arrangements for study leave and maternity leave.

(This list is not exhaustive.)

This research shows that district midwives in Nottingham maintained high caseloads with good outcomes. They worked in a defined geographical area and were not required to work in hospital; this kept travel and communication time to a minimum. However, there were difficulties in maintaining a proper balance of caseloads, a matter which was sometimes confounded by the midwives who were reluctant to give up clients. There is evidence that caseloads and workloads were monitored. The system failed in its lack of implementation of appropriate action to realign the caseloads, which would in turn have adjusted workloads.

Today, equitable caseloads could be ensured through systems where each midwife books an agreed number of women each month. However, this has inherent difficulties; for example, could this type of quota system restrict a woman's right to choose a midwife who had looked after her in a previous pregnancy or a midwife who lives near her because her monthly quota is full.

Ball *et al.* (1992) and Flint (1993) have produced some interesting calculations regarding caseloads. However, these would need to be considered in the context of the type of scheme chosen and the variables listed above. It seems obvious, however, that in a strictly domiciliary service the individual caseload potential is greater. All these issues need to be worked through carefully and in close liaison with practitioners, women and service providers.

CHOICE AND CONTROL FOR WOMEN

There is evidence that women in Nottingham were satisfied with the choices open to them, even though it is clear that they were siphoned into systems of care by two selection schemes, the first criteria led, the second streaming by social class. There is evidence that many socially dis-advantaged women did not get hospital beds and that women who knew that their medical or obstetric circumstances indicated a referral to hospital delayed or refrained from booking in order to ensure a home birth.

Indication that women welcomed the care of district midwives and the continuity they offered is evident in the fact that the majority of home-booked women had self-referred to a midwives' clinic without attempting to secure a hospital bed. Similarly, they returned to their midwife time and again. The value women set upon continuity of carer through labour and into the 'lying-in' period is indicated by the fact that many of them chose to continue with postnatal care from the midwife who had delivered them. This would have been a midwife they knew.

The truth regarding women's choice of place of birth, then and now, probably lies somewhere between two substantive research projects undertaken in Nottingham, almost 20 years apart. In his medical disser-tation, *A Survey of Home and Hospital Confinements in Nottingham*, Goodacre (1974), drawing upon earlier data, concluded that:

> Although it is generally the case that obstetric 'high risk' cases tend to be selected for hospital this is not always so; the mothers own prefer-ence and social conditions are sometimes found to outweigh some types of 'high risk' characteristic in determining the place of confine-ment, and opinion as to whether or not this is desirable varies greatly.
>
> Certainly the mothers in Nottingham seem generally to be con-fined where they would want to be and are mostly satisfied with the care received wherever their confinement was.
>
> *(Goodacre 1974: 139)*

Nearly 20 years later, in a culture which condemned home birth as irresponsible, from a survey of 1074 women following hospital birth in Nottingham, 27% said they wished they had been given information at booking about home birth (Allison 1991). It is likely that these women responded in the way they did because of dissatisfaction with the lack of choice available. Nevertheless, there is a clear message for the providers of future maternity services.

During the years of the study, there were only two NHS choices: home or hospital. Access to the hospital service was limited: women nevertheless had continuity of carer. During the period 1948 to 1968 a woman booking for delivery at the local maternity hospital might expect to see a maximum of 16 carers during her pregnancy, labour and postnatal period. She might expect to see only between two and four carers if booked for home, whereas in 1990 at the central maternity unit she was likely to see 40 carers throughout her pregnancy and birth (Allison 1991: 36–7).

THE BIRTH ENVIRONMENT

Attempts by providers over recent years to improve the hospital environment in which women give birth have been exciting. Indeed, schemes such as the 'Home from Home' project in Leicester and the midwifery-led unit in Bournemouth have been true innovations of our time and have provided choices for women which are exactly in line with those so frequently indicated in consumer surveys. In facilitating these changes, midwives have shown that they recognize the value of research and are prepared to respond to consumer opinion by reviewing their professional philosophical framework and adapting their practice.

Nevertheless, O'Brien (1978: 466) missed the point in arguing that a hospital birth environment needed to be improved to prevent women from 'voting with their feet' and insisting on home birth, whatever the risk. Likewise, conducting randomized controlled trials comparing birth room to labour ward experiences (Chapman et al. 1986: 182–7) in an attempt to identify the factor which makes women 'aesthetically' comfortable in labour are flawed at the outset. The purpose of the study was to recreate a 'home-like' environment as an obstetrically acceptable alternative to home birth. Every person's home is individual and different to the next and none are within a hospital. Each home gives its owner security of territory. An individual's territorial control is not transmutable, thus it can never be possible to recreate a home-like atmosphere in a hospital environment. For those women who are determined upon a home birth, no hospital recreation will suffice. For those who simply want to enjoy home comforts in labour these innovations are purpose made.

Macvicar *et al.* (1993: 316–23) argue that homely units within maternity hospitals or birth centres (as in the USA) provide the best of both worlds: a homely atmosphere and safety. For some women the desire to give birth at home can never be fulfilled by an alternative hospital experience. For them, the issue is not about wallpaper, carpet, the lack of availability of equipment, but about being in control in one's own environment, giving birth in the marriage bed, being there with your children to reduce the trauma they experience as their place in the family is adjusted by the arrival of a sibling. It is about being the host to carers and visitors in your own environment and not the guest of the carer in an unfamiliar setting nor the captive audience of whichever visitors choose to come and see you. Some women simply do not like hospitals.

For women who share these sentiments, birth anywhere other than at home will always be second-best and whenever there are insufficient home-birth facilities and carers, home birth will continue to appear on the consumer's agenda.

COLLECTING DATA FROM THE PAST: AUDITING THE FUTURE

Until recent years, midwives carried out around 50% of all births in Britain unsupervised and mostly unattended by doctors. Contemporaneous notes were kept, the birth was recorded in the midwife's personal register and notified to the local Registrar of births. Unfortunately, midwives had neither the time, knowledge nor encouragement to audit their own work effectively; such analysis as was undertaken was invariably medically led.

Obstetricians lead the field in maternity-care research; indeed, audit of maternal and perinatal death have long been the order of the day. This audit has resulted in critical analysis of obstetric practice. In the developing maternity services midwives are already learning to undertake their own audit and analysis of practice which will ultimately lead to changes in service delivery as a direct result of midwife-led research. Such audit may apply to local data, teams within a service or individual midwives. Within this study, there is the example that the audit of the domiciliary midwifery service by midwives, as opposed to data collection, may have led to a different interpretation of the safety of domiciliary midwifery services. It is now apparent that many of these interpretations were open to question. The medical interpretation of the 1958 Perinatal Survey, which so demoralized the overburdened midwives, was to have profound effects on the future administration of maternity care.

At a more basic level from within this study, we can see that proper analysis of breast-feeding outcomes by individual midwives may have given insight into how to mitigate the massive swing away from breast-feeding which began in the 1960s. Similarly, development of audit tools to examine the mortality outcomes of babies born at home and hospital may have led to identification of the factors which apparently made birth at home as safe as birth in hospital for low birthweight babies.

New types of care systems must be clearly defined so that appropriate data collection is implemented and useful comparisons made and opportunities for rigorous research identified. In past years, births nationally have been identified under medical headings, i.e. GP or obstetrician births. Thus the role and responsibility of the midwife have been statistically subsumed within a medical framework. It is important that in the future, midwifery-led care is identified separately so that meaningful comparisons are made.

In many ways the data collection from which the findings of this study were drawn was sound. It was relevant to the activities being carried out, assiduously collected year-on-year in a uniform manner across Britain. Thus in theory it was possible to make comparisons between the two major providers of maternity care, the hospital and domiciliary services, in terms of birth outcomes. Information about low birthweight babies, the legitimacy of babies at birth and the age of mothers were all useful indicators of changing social conditions and needs.

The Medical Officer of Health was responsible for the annual publication of birth statistics and maternity outcomes. Under the auspices of the Chief Medical Officer, similar data were collected each year across Britain. Changing social circumstances and professional developments were acknowledged by increased data collection: for example, in the 1950s the MOH began to identify mothers by their country of origin.

In his Annual Report, the MOH made some qualitative and quantitative comparisons between one year and another. Tables and charts were given with comparative data for home and hospital births, but apparently no systematic or rigorous analysis attempted. Within the Annual Reports of the Medical Officer of Health, other aspects of the health and well-being of the local population were reported both descriptively and in statistical data. If proper interpretation of the data had been made and presented to the Peel Committee, it would have been difficult for the argument for 100% hospital beds on the grounds of safety for mother and baby to be sustained.

After the reorganization of the NHS in 1972, little systematic data collection or publication of maternity outcomes appears to have taken place until recently. The 1979 House of Commons *Perinatal and Neonatal Mortality Report* (HMSO 1980) recommended that less birth data should be recorded. In 1995 it is time to review the data we keep and ensure that it is relevant to the care being given and that interpretation of the outcomes is rigorously undertaken to ensure that the care we give is constantly monitored in the best interests of mothers and babies. In terms of data collection, early analysis and monitoring performances the role of the Supervisor of Midwives was and is vital.

SUPERVISION OF MIDWIVES

Supervision of midwives, designed for the protection of mothers and babies, was central to the framework of the 1902 Midwives Act and has undoubtedly been one of the strengthening and enabling forces of the profession over the years.

It is clear from the work and oral evidence of the Supervisors of Midwives in this study that they viewed their function in terms of protecting women and babies. They achieved this through supervised deliveries and nursings and comprehensive scrutiny of personal registers, labour notes and drug prescription. However, it is equally clear that through the discussion of critical incidents, the midwife was allowed the opportunity to develop her ability to critically examine her practice and to consider alternative approaches in the safe and facilitative environment of her own home. Such reflection upon practice is greatly valued today as a means of practice development and validation of the theory that underpins an individual's philosophy of care. It is clear that district midwives developed concepts to improve practice and efficiency, such as the introduction of district registers and encouraging each other to take on the postnatal care of women they delivered when 'on call' but who were not their booked clients. As indicated earlier, such women often showed a preference for postnatal care from the midwife who delivered their baby. There are many other examples of innovation that arose as a result of supervised practice.

Central to the effective work of these supervisors was their location in relation to the function of the local supervising authority (LSA) and their line of management. The locus of the LSA was the local authority, housed in the public health department. The offices of the Supervisors of Midwives were similarly located in the health department, in close proximity to the Medical Officer of Health. They reported to him on a regular basis and worked with him in compiling midwifery data for presentation in annual reports.

The location of district midwifery services in the heart of the community was central to their effectiveness. Supervisors regularly visited women and midwives in their homes, understanding at first hand the social, economic, racial and political context in which the mothers and babies were living in their area. Working directly to the Medical Officer of Health, whose range of responsibility included among other things housing, education and social services, she was best placed to understand the context in which women lived and midwives worked and be in a position to influence.

Today, directors of public health medicine act as the guardians of local public health and it seems imperative that in some way the liaison between Supervisors of Midwives and departments of public health are widened. Whether babies are born in hospital or delivered at home, home is where they will all be reared and a clearer understanding of the function of the Supervisor could facilitate improvement in maternal and child health.

THE WAY FORWARD: READY TO DELIVER

This project shows that apparently some 52% of women who had a home birth in Nottingham between 1948 and 1972 did not fulfil the criteria for normal birth given by the Ministry of Health in 1967. Nevertheless, the maternal and infant outcomes were good. Transfers from home to hospital were low: 8.6% of women were known to have been transferred in the antenatal period and an estimated 1.1% during or around the time of labour.

The time has come when a woman's wishes will be paramount in making decisions about the place of birth. Carers have a duty to offer every opportunity to ensure that her decision is well-informed with readily understood, research-based information. Home birth was part of the culture of society and, until 1970, district midwives who undertook home births felt secure in the knowledge that they performed an honourable task which could not be done better by anyone else. The outcomes from this project indicate that they may well have been right in their assumption. Arguments that hospital outcomes were alone in being adversely skewed by women not booked to give birth there has been challenged, as has the notion that women who delivered at home were generally 'low risk'.

Midwives should be encouraged in the knowledge that they are the carer best placed to give the care that the majority of women who are having a normal childbirth experience want and need, wherever the birth takes place. Dingwall, Rafferty and Webster (1988: 165) argue that there has been no 'golden age' of licensed midwifery in Britain and that the view of the midwife as an independent practitioner as opposed to a medical assistant is unsupported. This study brings to centre stage the role of the midwife in its fullest sense. It shows midwives at their best, providing a 24-hour-a-day, 365-days-a-year, door-to-door service for women, offering continuity of carer, expertise, safety and some measure of control: a locality based service in all senses and arguably the 'golden age' of midwifery.

Midwives of today who long to give the service that *Changing Childbirth* demands must take heart from this evidence and know that this type of care and way of working could be translated into today's terms, with appropriate caseloads, support mechanisms and dedicated peer groups working across the organizational barrier between hospital and home. The challenge is there and some midwives are beginning to find a more satisfying way of working, with differing work patterns and the bonus of knowing that they are giving women what they want. The onus on the leaders of the profession is to ensure that midwives are given the proper support to take on this role.

Midwife-led care for women with appropriate medical and obstetric histories, who choose hospital or home birth, is one way in which the demands of today's maternity service policy is being met. For those who still harbour doubts about midwives' ability to deliver the care required for the future, the message of this study is simple: we have done it before.

However, todays' society is not comparable to that of yesterday. Family structures have changed, the number of children per family has reduced and women expect to have a career outside of their domestic life.Whilst housing, labour-saving appliances and home entertainment have improved for the majority, employment opportunities and job insecurity bring a different sort of stress into the homes of today's families.

Current policy directs that today's maternity service must be sensitive to the wishes of todays' women. If purchasers interpret guidance sensitively, then career opportunities for midwives will mirror women's choices for place of birth and carer. Whilst there is a need for some midwives to work more flexibly, the need for that strong core of hospital-based midwives who wish to give care to women who are more likely to be experiencing difficult pregnancies and births and those who choose hospital care has never been greater.

Local authority domiciliary midwifery services and the district midwives who provided home deliveries existed for 24 years under the NHS. It is 23 years since those services were disbanded and still the image of 'the district midwife' has consonance with notions of professionalism, service and autonomy. To some of today's midwives this is inspiring; to others it is an anathema.

At this moment of writing, some midwives have already found ways to give care to childbearing women which fulfil the expectations of *Changing Childbirth* and at the same time give them the type of job satisfaction they have never known before. Others are still searching or waiting for the way forward to become evident.

The good news is that the three professional organizations, the Royal College of Midwives, the Royal College of Obstetricians and Gynaecologists and the Royal College of General Practitioners, who will provide direction for the future maternity services agree that all proposals to change maternity services should take account of user views. Among many recommendations, they have agreed that home birth is an acceptable option for which appropriate information should be provided (Chamberlain and Patel 1994: 298).

Finally, there is a lesson to be learned about midwives' working conditions. The midwives who were interviewed remembered their time 'on the district' with affection because of the position they held in society and personal job satisfaction. Nevertheless, they were overworked, working hours which were not only unsocial but dangerous to their health. These women truly subjugated their domestic and social life to the needs of the domiciliary midwifery service. In reality, the service was run on the goodwill of the midwives and their families. For them, life was not all work and sleep – it was all work. History must not be repeated.

References

Allison, J. (1989) *The Changing Pattern of British Midwifery Practice 1936–1989*. Dissertation submitted in partial fulfilment of the MA in Social Policy and Administration, University of Nottingham.

Allison, J. (1991) *Report to the District General Manager Regarding the Future of the Midwifery Service*, Nottingham Health Authority.

Allison, J. (1993) Prematurity and Low Birthweight: An Alternative Management, in *Encyclopaedia of Childbearing: Critical Perspectives*, (ed. B.K. Rothman), Oryx Press, Phoenix, Arizona, USA.

Ball, J.A., Flint, C., Garvey, M., Jackson Baker, A. and Page, L. *et al.* (1992) *Who's left Holding The Baby?*, Nuffield Institute, University of Leeds.

Brown, D. (1965) *The General Practitioner in Obstetrics*. Maternal and Child Health, December, London.

Burnell, J., McCarthy, M., Chamberlain, G.U.P., Hawkins, D.F. and Elbourne, D. (1982) Patient Preference and Postnatal Hospital Stay. *Journal of Obstetrics and Gynaecology*, **3**.

Butler, N.R. and Bonham, D.G. (1963) *Perinatal Mortality*, Livingstone, Edinburgh and London.

Campbell, R., Macdonald, Dav, Macfarlane, A. and Beral (1984) Home Births in England and Wales: 1979: Perinatal Death According to Intended Place of Delivery. *British Medical Journal*, **289**.

Campbell, R. and Macfarlane, A. (1987, reprinted 1994) *Where to be Born, the Debate and the Evidence,* NPEU, Oxford.

Caplan, M. and Madeley, R. (1985) *Home Deliveries in Nottingham 1980–1981*, Public Health, London, **99**.

Carter, G.B. and Dodds, G.H. (1953) *A Dictionary of Midwifery and Public Health*, Faber and Faber, London.

Chalmers, I., Enkin, M. and Keirse, M.J.N.C. (eds) (1989) *Effective Care in Pregnancy and Childbirth*, Oxford University Press, Oxford.

Chamberlain, G. and Patel, N. (eds) (1994) *The Future of the Maternity Services*, RCOG Press, London.

Chapman, M.G., Jones, M., and Spring, J.E. (1986) The Use of the Birthroom: a

Randomised Controlled Trial Comparing Delivery With That in The Labour Ward. *British Journal of Obstetrics and Gynaecology*, **93**.

City of Nottingham (1949–72) *Annual Reports of the Health Services*, Medical Officer of Health W. Dodd, MD.

CMB (1948) *Rules Framed by the Central Midwives Board*, 19th edn, Spottiswoode Ballantyne, London.

CMB (1950) *Rules of the Central Midwives Board*, 20th edn

CMB (1962) *Rules of the Central Midwives Board*, 25th edn

CMB (1963) *Suggestions and Instructions Regarding the Conduct of the Course of Training for Pupil Midwives*

CMB (1969) *The 23rd Report of the Central Midwives Board*

CMB (1971) *Suggestions and Instructions Regarding the Conduct of Training of Pupil Midwives*

Damstra-Wijmenga, S.M.I. (1984) Home Confinement: the Positive Results in Holland. *Journal of the Royal College of General Practitioners*, August, London.

Dingwall, R., Rafferty, A.M. and Webster, C. (1988) *An Introduction to the Social History of Nursing*, Routledge, Chapman & Hall, London.

DHSS (1973) *On the State of the Public Health: The Annual Report of the Chief Medical Officer of Health and Social Security for the Year 1972*, HMSO, London.

Flint, C. (1993) *Midwifery Teams and Caseloads*, Butterworth Heinemann, Oxford.

Goodacre, J. (1974) A Survey of Home and Hospital Confinements in Nottingham. A Dissertation for Part 2 of the Degree of Bachelor of Medical Science (Honours) Department of Community Health, University of Nottingham.

HMSO (1959) *Report of the Maternity Services Committee*, London.

HMSO (1967) *Safer Obstetric Care*, Oxford.

HMSO (1968) *Health Services and Public Health Act*, London.

HMSO (1969) *Local Government Reform Report of the Royal Commission on Local Government in England*, London.

HMSO (1970) *Domiciliary Midwifery and Maternity Bed Needs*, London.

HMSO (1972) *Management Arrangements for the Reorganised NHS*, London.

HMSO (1972) *National Health Service Reorganisation*, London.

HMSO (1974) *Present Day Practice in Infant Feeding*, London.

HMSO (1976) *Priorities for Health and Personal Social Services in England: A Consultative Document*, London.

HMSO Social Services Committee (1979/1980) *Perinatal and Neonatal Mortality, 2nd Report from the Social Services Committee Session*, London.

HMSO (1989) *Women's Experience of Maternity Care: A Survey Manual*, London.

HMSO (1991) *House of Commons: All Party Select Committee into the Maternity Services*, London.

HMSO (1993) *Changing Childbirth Part 1 and Part 2 Report of the Expert Maternity Group*, London.

Macvicar, J. *et al.* (1993) Simulated Home Delivery in Hospital: A Randomised Controlled Trial. *British Journal of Obstetrics and Gynaecology*, April, **100**, pp. 316–23.

Maggs, (1994) *Direct But Different: Executive Summary*, Crown Publication, Maggs Research Associates.

Marwick, A. (1970/1989) *The Nature of History*, Macmillan Education, London.

Mason, D. (1963) *Some Aspects of the Work of the Midwife*, Nursing Research Committee, National Florence Nightingale Memorial Committee, London.

Maternity Alliance (1993/4) *Annual Report of the Maternity Alliance*, London.

Midwives Chronicle and Nursing Notes (1967) *Viewpoint*, p. 416, December, London.

Munro, A. (1982/3) *Maternity Care in Action: Parts 1/2/3*. Reports of the Maternity Services Advisory Committee, HMSO, London.

Murphy, J.F., Daumey, MN., Gray, O.P. and Chalmers, I. (1984) Planned and unplanned deliveries at home: implications of a changing ratio. *British Medical Journal*, **288**.

NAO (1990) *Maternity Services, Report by the Comptroller and Auditor General*, National Audit Office, HMSO, London.

Newson, J. and Newson, E. (1963/1974) *Patterns of Infant Care in an Urban Community*, Penguin Books, Middlesex.

Nottingham Evening News (1964) *Midwives Register a Protest*, December, Nottingham.

Oakley, A. (1984/6) *The Captured Womb*, Basil Blackwell, Oxford.

O'Brien, M. (1978) Home and Hospital: A Comparison of the Experiences of Mothers Having Home and Hospital Confinements. *Journal of the Royal College of General Practitioners*, August.

Stearn, R.H. (1968) The Place of Domiciliary Midwifery, in *Midwives Chronicle and Nursing Notes*, November.

Tew, M. (1978) Intended Place of Delivery and Perinatal outcome. *British Medical Journal*, **1**, 1139–40.

Tew, M. (1979) The Safest Place of Birth. *Lancet*, **i**, 1388–90.

Tew, M. (1985) Place of Birth and Perinatal Mortality. *Journal of the Royal College of General Practitioners*, **35**.

Tew, M. (1986) Do Obstetric Intranatal Interventions Make Birth Safer? *British Journal of Obstetrics and Gynaecology*, **93**, 659–74.

Tew, M. (1995) *Safer Childbirth*, 2nd edn, Chapman & Hall, London.

Tew, M. and Damstra-Wijmenga, S.M.I. (1991) Safest Birth Attendants: Recent Dutch Evidence. *Midwifery*, **7**, Longman, Harlow.

Towler, J. and Bramall, J. (1986) *Midwives in History and Society*, Croom Helm, London.

Tyler, S. (1994) Maternity Care and the Paradox of Plenty. *British Journal of Midwifery*, **2**, 11.

UKCC *Handbook of Midwives Rules*, UKCC, London.

Van Alten, D., Eskes, M. and Treffers, P.E. (1989) Midwifery in The Netherlands: The Wormerveer Study: Selection, Mode of Delivery, Perinatal Mortality and Infant Morbidity. *British Journal of Obstetrics and Gynaecology*, **96**.

Wedge, P. and Prosser, H. (1973) *Born To Fail*, Arrow Books, London.

Wraight, A., Ball, J., Seccombe, I. and Stockli, J. (1993) *Mapping Team Midwifery*, A Report to the Department of Health, IMS, Brighton.

Appendix A City of Nottingham instructions to midwives (1957)

SUGGESTED
TIME TABLE

Morning
: Nursings to be commenced at 9am when possible. Attendance at antenatal clinics.

Afternoon
: Antenatal visits, doctor's clinics and relaxation classes. One afternoon or evening to be kept free for patients to attend the midwife's house for booking and advice.

Evening
: Nursing visits to be made for three days after delivery for normal cases and otherwise for as long as necessary, e.g. sutured perineum, illness or abnormality of mother or child.

Urgent calls

When the midwife is out, a notice must be placed on the door showing the whereabouts of the midwife, and an approximate time at each address.

Off duty

By arrangement with the relieving midwife and the Supervisor of Midwives.

Holidays

Five weeks annually; the leave year starts on 1st April. (Author's note: This included Bank Holiday.)

Booking

At the time of booking, the mother should be urged to attend either her General Practitioner or welfare centre. The leaflet *Preparation for Home Confinement* should be given and explained, also full information regarding analgesia and maternity packs. The patient should be instructed to notify the midwife before 9 am if she is likely to need her during the morning.

Antenatal

Mothers should be seen and examined at regular intervals, especially during the last two months of pregnancy. Defaulters must be followed up.

ANALGESIA

Gas and air or Trilene

A certificate of fitness given by the booked GP or welfare centre medical officer must be obtained. A third person must be present during administration. For midwives without cars, gas and air machines are kept at the City Transport offices, tel. 45745, and are delivered on request during confinement to the patient's home; immediately after confinement, they must arrange for the collection of the machine by the City Transport staff.

Notification cards

Both a pink and a white card should be completed for each birth and posted to the Health Department within 24 hours of the confinement. Pink cards only to be completed for miscarriages and emergency calls, whether or not the baby is delivered by the midwife.

Pethidine

This is supplied through the Health Department (it comes under the Dangerous Drugs regulation) and each midwife must show her own drug book and file of cases booked, in order to obtain each supply.

Medical aid forms

When medical aid has been sought, a copy of the medical aid form should be sent to the Health Department within 24 hours. All the particulars asked for should be completed, including the time of sending for the doctor. For procedure in calling for Doctor, see *Handbook of CMB*, page 84. Where the doctor was booked for Maternity Medical Services, this should be stated on the medical aid form by the initials MMS.

Stillbirths

Where the midwife is present at birth and the child has shown no signs of life, or when the birth is unattended and the baby is macerated or deformed, the stillbirth form should be completed and sent to the Health Department. The registrar's form should be completed and given to the nearest relative to take to the Registrar of Births, who will give a certificate for burial.

Where the midwife is not present at the birth and the child is not macerated, or deformed, medical aid should be sought at once. Otherwise the case must be reported to the coroner.

ABORTIONS AND MISCARRIAGES

The midwife must attend when sent for and call in medical aid in accordance with CMB Rules, or ask for admission to hospital if necessary. If the patient is kept at home she must be nursed for ten days.

ANTEPARTUM HAEMORRHAGE, POSTPARTUM HAEMORRHAGE, PREMATURE LABOUR

If the midwife considers hospital treatment is essential and she is not able to contact the doctor, she should telephone the duty registrar at the City Hospital direct, tel. 63361. The District Flying Squad is based at the City Hospital, and in an emergency the midwife can call it out herself.

OPHTHALMIA NEONATORUM AND LESSER EYE INFECTION

Medical aid should be sought for all infants with inflammation or discharge from the eyes, however slight.The appropriate form should be filled in and sent at once to this department for follow-up visits.

PYREXIA

Any rise of temperature necessitating the calling of medical aid *(Handbook of CMB Rules,* page 83) should be reported at once to the Supervisor of Midwives.

PEMPHIGUS

Any suspicious blisters or spots should be reported immediately to the Supervisor of Midwives and instructions obtained. A form of notification of 'liability to be a source of infection' must be sent to this department in accordance with CMB rules.

ARTIFICIAL FEEDING

In all cases where breast-feeding cannot be carried out, the midwife must notify this department on the appropriate form. It is expected that a midwife will do her utmost to promote breast-feeding and will encourage patients to prepare their breasts during pregnancy.

NOTIFICATION OF DEATH OF MOTHER OR CHILD

Particulars to be telephoned to this department as soon as possible and the appropriate form completed.

MATERNITY PACKS

These are available for all patients nursed at home.The one to be used at confinement, No. 203, contains sanitary pads, cord dressings, ties and powder, cotton wool, a sheet of tarred paper and an accouchement sheet; the last named is to be used as a sterile towel under the patient at the time of delivery.

Smaller packs are provided for miscarriages (No. 205) and patients discharged from hospital (No. 204) for home nursing.

MASKS

A clean mask is to be worn at each visit to the patient, whether during labour or for nursing. Used masks to be carried in a separate bag, in the outer pocket of the nursing bag. Each midwife is responsible for laundering her own masks.

DELIVERY GOWNS

A gown and cap must be worn for each delivery and nursing. They should be kept suitably wrapped in the patient's rooms.

WEEKLY REPORT

The form to be completed and returned to this department by first post on Monday morning.

DRUGS AND OTHER REQUISITES

These are obtainable from the Health Department when the midwife visits on Wednesday or Thursday afternoons, between 2.30 and 4.30 pm.

A midwife is allowed to use certain drugs on her own responsibility (see *Handbook of CMB*, page 80).

The following are supplied by this department:

Antiseptics

Dettol; use $2\frac{1}{2}\%$ strength, or 1–40, by diluting $\frac{1}{2}$ oz dettol to pint water.
Methylated spirits.
Milton (premature baby nursings only).

Stimulants

Cardiac
Coramine, by i.m. injection to mother dose 2 c.c.
by i.m injection to baby $\frac{1}{2}$ c.c.

Respiratory
Lobeline for asphyxiated babies after clearing air passages, dose 1 ampoule, i.e. 3mgm intramuscularly.

Ergot

Ergometrine by intramuscular injection 0.5 mgm. may be repeated once immediately.

Ergot prep (gr. $2\frac{1}{2}$) orally tabs i or ii after delivery for suitable cases where ergometrine is not necessary.

Sedatives and analgesics

Pethidine, 1 ampoule, i.e. 100 mgm., may be repeated once every four hours.

Mist. Pot. Brom. and Chloral (grs × åå in 1 drachm) dose II drachms orally.

Gas and Air

Trilene

Other

Synkavit, imi for mother during labour

10 MGM ampoules

imi for baby, 1 mgm. ampoules

April 1957

11/G

Appendix B Glossary and abbreviations

Accouchement sheet (see Appendix A) A small disposable sheet supplied in the delivery pack, used as a sterile towel under the patient's buttocks at delivery (see illustration on page 80).

Ascites An accumulation of free fluid in the peritoneal cavity, a condition rarely seen in pregnancy.

Anencephaly Failure of development of the brain and cranium.

Antenatal clinic (ANC) (in the context of this project) A clinic for the examination and supervision of pregnant women conducted by the local health authority under Section 22 of the NHS Act 1946.

Antepartum haemorrhage Bleeding from the genital tract anytime from the 28th week of pregnancy until the child is born.

Asphyxia neonatorum Failure of child to breathe at birth.

BBA (in the context of the project) Born at home before the arrival of the district midwife.

Central Midwives Board (CMB) The statutory, regulating body for midwives in England and Wales from 1902 to 1983.

Certificate of expected confinement Certificate issued by a midwife or doctor at or after the 26th week of pregnancy which allowed the patient to claim the maternity grant, allowance and other maternity benefits.

City midwives (in the context of this project) Refers to district midwives employed by the City of Nottingham Medical Officer of Health. Similarly, those midwives who were employed by the County of Nottingham Medical Officer of Health were described as county midwives.

Coramine (see Appendix A) A proprietary preparation of nikethamide (a cardiac and respiratory stimulant). Occasionally used on the mother in the case of collapse, and for the new-born in cases of severe asphyxia neonatorum.

Direct entrant (see also midwifery training) Sometimes referred to as single certificate midwife; a midwife who had entered midwifery training without previous nurse training.

District midwife The term introduced by the Rushcliffe Report (1948) to replace terms previously used for the category of domiciliary midwife, i.e. county midwife, borough midwife, municipal midwife.

District register (sometimes called area register) A register kept by a partnership of midwives, usually filled in at the booking clinic which contained details of all women in an area booked for home birth. Over time, the midwives would record what happened to the patients, e.g. transferred to hospital booking, delivered at home, miscarried and who gave the care.

Double duty nurse/worker A term to describe women who worked on the district as a district nurse and midwife. Frequently employed in rural areas.

Drawer sheet A narrow cotton sheet placed across the middle of the bed, over the bottom sheet, as in hospital beds.

Eclampsia (in the context of this project) A severe degree of toxaemia characterised by fits. Life-threatening to mother and fetus.

Ergometrine (see Appendix A) Oxytocic drug, used after delivery for retained placenta and control of haemorrhage.

Expected date of delivery (EDD) Calculated by adding nine calendar months and seven days to the date of the last normal period, in a woman who has a regular 28-day menstrual cycle.

Executive committee A council established by Section 31 of the NHS Act

1946, for the area of a local health authority, providing general medical, dental pharmaceutical and supplementary ophthalmic service for such area. Superseded by the Family Practitioner Committee.

Family Practitioner Committee (FPC) See above.

Foetus Old form of spelling of fetus.

Gas and air An inhalation analgesic mixture of nitrous oxide and air.

General Practitioner (GP)

General practitioner obstetrician (GPO) A GP whose named appeared on the obstetric list.

Gestation Pregnancy: understood to mean number of weeks duration of a pregnancy.

Gestational diabetes Glucose intolerance appearing during pregnancy.

Grande multipara A woman of high parity. Usually one who has borne four or more children.

Gravid Pregnant.

Gravida A woman who is pregnant. Hence gravida one, a woman who is pregnant for the first time.

Intrauterine fetal death (IUFD) Death of the fetus in utero, generally used in reference to a death which occurs in pregnancy rather than labour.

Independent midwife (in the context of this project) A midwife who continued to practise in a self-employed capacity after the implementation of the National Health Service, when the majority of domiciliary midwives became local government employees.

Liquor (amnii) The fluid which fills the amniotic sac, in the uterus, in which the fetus floats.

Lobeline (see Appendix A) A respiratory stimulant, used to treat asphyxia neonatorum.

Local authority (LA) Local government.

Local supervising authority (LSA) The authority designated to undertake the statutory supervision of midwives, according to the Rules (after 1974: the Regional Health Authority. Prior to 1974: the Local Health Authority).

Low birthweight (LBW) Babies weighing 5lb 8oz or less at birth.

Macerated fetus A fetus which is born with skin and superficial tissue peeling off. Evidence that intrauterine death had occurred at least some hours before birth.

Malpresentation Any presentation of the fetus other than the vertex.

Maternity grant A cash grant payable to a woman on her own or her husband's insurance, whether or not the child was born alive. The grant was paid in respect of each child born, thus it would be doubled in the case of twins if they were both alive after 12 hours. In 1953 the grant was £4; in 1969 it was £22.

Midwifery training Previously in two parts, undertaken in two different training schools. Part 1 concentrated on theory and practical hospital experience, while the six-month Part 2 focused on public health issues and the adaptation of the pupil to 'district midwifery'. Certificates were given by the CMB for the successful completion of each part (CMB 1963).

Medical Officer (MO) (of a local authority antenatal clinic) Generally required to have been qualified for three years and to have had adequate experience of practical midwifery and antenatal work.

Medical Officer of Health (MOH) Chief Executive Officer of the Local Authority, Health/Public Health Department (qualifications: registered medical practitioner, registered diploma in public health). Required to present an annual report to his council.

Membrane sweep (or stripping the membranes) Sweeping the membranes from the lower uterine segment during vaginal examination at term. Used as a means of inducing labour.

Mist. pot. brom. and chloral (see Appendix A) Mixture of potassium bromide and chloral hydrate. A powerful hypnotic drug, causing sleep, used in the first stage of labour.

Multigravida A woman pregnant for the second or subsequent time.

Multiparous A woman who has delivered more than one baby.

National Health Service (NHS) Act 1946 Provided for the establishment of a comprehensive health service for England and Wales.

Neonatal death (NND) A death within 28 days of birth.

Ophthalmia neonatorum (see Appendix A) Conjunctivitis in the child, occurring within 21 days of birth and notifiable as ophthalmia neo-natorum.

Parity The number of children a woman has borne.

Patch A geographical area for which a district midwife had responsibility for all aspects of domiciliary birth, whether the women were booked for home birth or not.

Pemphigus (see Appendix A) Bullous impetigo: pemphigus occurring in infants. Extremely infectious and contagious. The midwife was required to report any occurrence of watery blisters in the new-born, whatever the apparent cause.

Perinatal mortality rate (PNMR) The number of stillbirths, plus the number of deaths occurring during the first week of life per 1000 total births, i.e. live and stillbirths.

Personal register (in the context of this project) The register, kept by the midwife, which was a chronologically ordered and contemporaneously kept account of every delivery she undertook.

Pethidine (see Appendix A) Analgesic, antispasmodic drug (controlled by Dangerous Drugs Act) administered to women in labour by intramuscular injection.

Pupil midwife (PM) Old term for midwives in training.

Postnatal After childbirth.

Postpartum After labour.

Postpartum haemorrhage (PPH) (in the context of this project) Bleeding from the vagina of more than 20 ounces (500 ml) after the delivery of the baby.

Premature labour By an internationally adopted standard (World Health

Assembly, 1948) a premature baby was defined as one which, at birth, weighs 2500 grammes (5.5lb) or less.

Primigravida A woman pregnant for the first time.

Primipara A woman who has given birth to her first child.

Primiparous Having borne one child.

Retained placenta When the normal process of separation and/or expulsion of the placenta during the third stage of labour has failed.

Roll of midwives Every candidate who was successful in the Second Examination (Part 2) had her name entered on the Roll of Midwives, maintained by the Central Midwives Board.

Royal College of Midwives (RCM) (in the context of this project) The professional association of midwives; formerly the Incorporated Midwives' Institute, founded in 1881. Principal aim, 'to raise the efficiency and improve the status of midwives' (Carter and Dobbs 1953: 638).

Rushcliffe Committees Committees set up by the Minister of Health in 1941/1942, the Nurses Salaries Committee and the Midwives Salaries Committee, under the chairmanship of Lord Rushcliffe. Replaced under Section 66 of the NHS Act 1946 by the Whitley Machinery.

Single certificate midwife (See direct entrant.)

Sparklets apparatus Oxygen apparatus issued to district midwives.

Special care unit (SCU) Units designed for the particular care of low birthweight and sick babies, now superceded by neonatal intensive care units.

State certified midwife (SCM) Old title given to midwives who had successfully completed Parts 1 and 2 of their midwifery training.

Stillbirth (SB) (in the context of this project) A child which has issued from its mother after the 28th week of pregnancy and which did not at any time after having been completely expelled show any sign of life. (NB: the definition was revised in October 1992.)

Synkavit (see Appendix A) Synthetic vitamin K: given to mothers in labour for the prevention of haemorrhagic disease of the newborn, or to affected babies as curative treatment.

Tarred sheet (see Appendix A) A sheet of tarred paper (waterproofed), supplied in the sterile maternity pack, which was placed under the accouchement sheet just before delivery (see illustration page 80).

Teaching district midwife A district midwife approved by the Central Midwives Board to teach pupil midwives during that part of their training which took place in the woman's own home (CMB 1962: 14).

Trilene (trichlorethylene) An analgesic vapour which was administered in labour through a special type of mask held in place by the mother.

Triple duty nurse/worker Used to describe women who took on the triple responsibilities of district nurse, midwife and health visitor, usually in remote rural areas.

Vandid (Vanillic acid diethylamide) 3 mg. was dropped on the infant's tongue to stimulate respiration at birth (da Cruz 1937 and 1967: 388).

Vertex (Vx) Area of the fetal head which is usually the part to appear first at the vulva during labour. A normal presentation.

Appendix C Abridged excerpts from a midwife's register

Abridged extract from the register of a City of Nottingham district midwife August/September (early 1960s)

Age	Date of Booking	EDC	Doctor booked	Called in emerg	Doctor present at Delivy	No. previo labours + misc	ANC given by a.Clinic b.Mlwife c.Doctor	Present-ation	Date & hour of infant birth	Birth weight	Sex of infant Alive or Dead	Condition of infant then breast fed complemented or supplemented	Remarks
24	9 June	10 Aug	yes	no	no	2	b c	vx	9 Aug	7.4	male live	breast satis	Normal delivery 3rd stage complete
30	16 June	30 Aug	no	no	no	2	b c	vx	12 Aug	6.0	female live	breast satis	Normal delivery 3rd stage complete
27	14 July	22 Aug	yes	no	no	3+1	b c	vx	12 Aug	7.4	male live	breast satis	Normal delivery 3rd stage complete
30	17 Feb	2 Aug	yes	no	no	1	b c	vx	17 Aug	8.0	female live	breast satis	Normal delivery 3rd stage complete
45	unbookd for home bkd CHN	23 Aug	yes	no	no	16	hospital	?	20 Aug	7.8	male live	nursed CHN	Normal delivery BBA 3rd stage complete mother/baby satis-admitted CHN
29	28 April	16 Aug	yes	no	no	2	b c	vx	23 Aug	8.4	female live	Art.t satis	Normal delivery 3rd stage complete
26	31 July	15 Aug	no	no	no	0	b	vx	24 Aug	8.4	female live	breast satis	Normal delivery 3rd stage complete
24	17 April	8 Sept	yes	no	no	0	b c	vx	27 Aug	7.12	male live	breast satis	Normal delivery 3rd stage complete
17	28 Feb	3 Sept	yes	no	no	0	b c	vx	5 Sept	7.8	male live	breast satis	Normal delivery 3rd stage complete
20	19 April	24 Sept	yes	no	no	2	b c	face	5 Sept	6.0	female live	Art satis	Face presentation 3rd stage complete
16	20 Feb	28 Sept	yes	no	no	0	b c	vx	5 Sept	6.0	male live	breast satis	Normal delivery 3rd stage complete
31	10 April	15 Sept	yes	no	no	5	b	vx	12 Sept	8.0	male live	Art satis	Normal delivery 3rd stage complete
19	unbookd	?	no	yes	no	0	c	vx	12 Sept	1.8	female dead	SB anenceph	Called 5.5 am, Dr called.Normal delivery macerated anencephalic foetus 3rd stage complete Mother satis
42	18 June	End Sept	yes	no	no	2	b c	vx	13 Sept	10.12	female live	breast satis	Normal delivery 3rd stage complete

Vx = Vertex (normal, head first, delivery); CHN = City Hospital Nottingham; Anencephalic = congenital abnormality

Appendix D Unexplored aspects of the study

The City of Nottingham district midwives' registers and Medical Officer of Health reports have formed the main data source for this book. Some have now been returned to the midwives who lent them for the purpose of this study. However, there still remains a cache of material which has been gifted and which will be catalogued in the Royal College of Midwives archive when the refurbishing of RCM headquarters is complete. This material as a data source remains largely unexplored.

The following is an account of that material and an overview of some of the issues that could be researched when the data becomes available.

AVAILABLE MATERIAL

District/area registers for City of Nottingham

Contain information about all women in a geographical area who were booked for care with a partnership of midwives. Probably 100 registers containing 25 000 entries.

District midwives' personal registers from other areas, 1929–72

Contents as above. Information contained in approximately 30 registers. Approximately 5000 births.

Pupil midwives' casebooks

It was a requirement of training that pupil midwives kept a casebook register of ten of the women they delivered. There are 12 casebooks covering the period 1945 to 1972.

Personal registers of hospital-based midwives 1946–62

District midwives' drug books

Approximately 20 books. Contents:

- type and amount of drugs issued to individual midwives;
- record of doses to individual women.

Medical aid books

Contain occasions on which midwives summoned medical aid by cause.

Official lists of names and addresses of district midwives

For City of Nottingham for 1956, 1957, 1958, 1969, 1971, 1972, 1974. Contents:

- names and addresses of midwives;
- area in which they worked;
- name and address of their partners;
- list of premature baby midwives and relief midwives;
- name of Supervisor of Midwives.

Interviews

Ten district midwives, three hospital midwives, two GPOs and two Supervisors have been interviewed.

Midwives' off duties, holiday lists, diaries, stationery, letters, policies, procedures, photographs, newspaper cuttings, unpublished record books and data collected by Supervisors of Midwives

Various memorabilia collected from retired district midwives

Uniforms, equipment, gas and air machines, watches, nursing bags and contents, textbooks, mothercraft books, ration books, etc.

POSSIBLE AREAS TO EXPLORE
(including those that remain unexplored from the data used in this book).

The following list of possible areas for research is not exhaustive; some of the issues have particular relevance today:

Perinatal deaths by cause and number for home and hospital, circumstance, amount of antenatal care and place in the family.

Pupils by number of deliveries attended by midwife or GPO or alone, by outcome.

Cost of the service some costings of the domiciliary midwifery service are possible, by comparison over time.

Drugs all drugs used by district midwives are recorded, interesting retrospective studies are possible. Records include:

- pethidine;
- oxytocic drugs;
- neonatal stimulants;
- gas and air;
- trichlorethylene;
- vitamin K;
- local anaesthetic.

Perineal outcomes incidence of perineal damage and episiotomy can be assessed by midwife, by year.

Labour a number of issues related to labour can be researched, including:

- length of labour by outcome;
- outcome of labour by attendant;
- outcome of labour by time of arrival of attendant;
- outcome of labour by gestation at booking;
- outcome of labour by parity;
- outcome of labour by age;
- outcome by drugs in labour.

Abnormal births outcome of abnormal or high risk cases delivered at home could be assessed, including:

- breech births;
- multiple births;
- abnormal presentations;
- GP and obstetrician inductions at home.

This is simply an example of some of the many issues related to birth at home which could be systematically researched from the available data.

Appendix E

POLITICAL AND ORGANIZATIONAL HISTORY OF NHS DISTRICT MIDWIFERY
1948–1972

STATUTE/REPORT YEAR	SOME FINDINGS/RECOMMENDATIONS/ POLICY	EFFECT ON DOMICILIARY SERVICE
Midwives Act 1936	LSAS required to provide a service of full-time salaried midwives for home confinements. Independent midwives were either brought into the service or paid off by the authority. A few remained in independent practice. LSAs could employ midwives themselves or contract those from voluntary associations and welfare councils. Standard working conditions were not laid down.	Midwives of the Queens Institute of District Nursing, who practised good domiciliary midwifery, especially in the rural counties and a very large proportion of the independent midwives in 'serious' practice, joined with others to provide a suitable service under the new conditions. The new domiciliary midwives continued to practise as individuals, carrying their own caseload.
National Health Service Act 1946	Amplified the 1936 Midwives Act. Independent practice not ended but LSAs required to employ domiciliary midwives, or to make arrangements to use hospital district practices. Maternity services organized under tripartite administration of the hospital authorities, the local executive councils (representing GPs) and the local health authorities for domiciliary midwifery services. Women were entitled to book the services of both midwife and GP which caused confusion about the role of the midwife and GP, leading to the 1949 Government Working Party statement that the doctor is the midwife's partner ... and no mere 'delivery woman'.	The organization of domiciliary midwifery services across Britain was similar to that described in this document for Nottingham. The major difference was between the staffing and organization of city and rural areas. In the latter there was a greater use of double and triple workers. District midwives worked as individual, caseload-carrying practitioners, within partnerships or groups. There was no professional or pay hierarchy. They undertook consultations in their own homes or clinics and increasingly became car-users.

STATUTE/REPORT YEAR	SOME FINDINGS/RECOMMENDATIONS/ POLICY	EFFECT ON DOMICILIARY SERVICE
NHS Amendment 1949	LSAS required to render all services reasonably necessary for proper care of women, e.g. analgesia.	Over the next few years all domiciliary midwives were issued with gas and air, pethidine and oxygen.
Working Party on Midwives Report 1949	Compulsory appointment of non-medical Supervisors of midwives (single certificate midwives not debarred), to work directly under the medical Administrative Officer (usually the Medical Officer of Health).	Domiciliary midwifery services were professionally and managerially led by an 'expert' in maternity care.
Committee of Enquiry Into the Cost of the NHS (Guillebaud Report) 1955	The tripartite structure of administering the maternity services was noted to be causing difficulty and confusion. In some places GPs were staffing local authority clinics on a sessional basis. Lack of clarity on who paid for services of GP in an emergency when the GP had not undertaken to give care.	Some cross-functional confusion; district midwives were frequently the only carer at local authority clinics. In some areas they also worked as unpaid clinic nurses at GP surgeries.
Report of the Maternity Services Committee (Cranbrook Report) 1959	Amplified findings of Guillebaud regarding confusion caused by tripartite administration of maternity services. Committee found that uneven provision of maternity services across the country meant that some women who wanted hospital birth were unable to secure a bed, and some women who were high risk were insisting on home confinement. In terms of cost, hospital confinement was found to be more expensive to the state, and cheaper to the woman. Complaints of 'casual' treatment and loss of dignity were made about institutional birth. Committee found that the benefits of home delivery outweighed the slight risk of unforeseen complications.	Some women were receiving care from the local authority clinic, GP and district midwife. Domiciliary midwives were still delivering and giving total care to 35% of annual births; percentage varied across the country. In Nottingham it remained at 50% until the 1960s. Some district midwives were already complaining of loss of role and identity as birth moved into hospital and their primary role became that of caring for hospital-delivered women postnatally. Fragmentation of care and loss of continuity of known carer at birth and control affected women and midwives.

STATUTE/REPORT YEAR	SOME FINDINGS/RECOMMENDATIONS/ POLICY	EFFECT ON DOMICILIARY SERVICE
Local Government Reform 1969	England should be divided into 61 new local government areas. A single authority will be responsible for all personal social services, opening the way for the development of a comprehensive service for families and individuals	With the demise of the old local authorities, by the early 1970s the newly formed health authorities organized the community midwifery services to undertake two functions: to provide community midwives as members of primary health care teams, led by GPs and to give a fragmented antenatal and postnatal service to women booked for hospital delivery. By 1980 home births were less than 1% of total births in Britain.
Domiciliary Midwifery and Maternity Bed Needs (Peel Report) 1970	Increased appreciation among profession and public that confinement in hospital is the safest arrangement, irrespective of considerations of cost of convenience. 'Discussion on advantages or disadvantages of home or hospital confinement are in one sense academic.' Recommendation for 100% hospital birth on grounds of safety.	Together with the Local Government Reform, the Peel Report saw the end of district midwifery as a discrete service offering a home birth with continuity of carer and women's choice and control.
Management Arrangements for the Reorganized NHS 1972	Multi-disciplinary management teams formed at each level to plan and co-ordinate health services jointly.	Loss of separate identity for midwives within the NHS as an individual and unique profession, whose responsibilities require self-management and pro-fessional control.

Index

NOTES

NOTES